Stop Stressing Me Out:
7 Solutions to Overcome Overwhelm & Conquer Disease *Naturally*

Dr. Lisa Lewis, ND, LAc.

Copyright © 2013 Dr. Lisa Lewis, ND, LAc All rights reserved. No portion of this book may be reproduced mechanically, electronically, or by any other means, including photocopying, without written permission of the publisher. It is illegal to copy this book, post it to a website, or distribute it by any other means without permission from the publisher.

Limits of Liability and Disclaimer of Warranty

The author and publisher shall not be liable for your misuse of this material. This book is strictly for informational and educational purposes.

Warning – Disclaimer

The purpose of this book is to educate and entertain. The author and/or publisher do not guarantee that anyone following these techniques, suggestions, tips, ideas, or strategies will become successful. The author and/or publisher shall have neither liability nor responsibility to anyone with respect to any loss or damage caused, or alleged to be caused, directly or indirectly by the information contained in this book.

ISBN: 978-0-9890977-0-3

Get your free "Stop Stressing Me Out" quiz!

"More Information and More Insight: 3 Ways to Release Your Stress Even Faster"

Take the quiz and you will:

1. See how high (or, hopefully, low) you score on the "Stop Stressing Me Out" quiz. Find out how much stress you really have.

2. Discover the physical signs and symptoms associated with stress, which signs and symptoms you have, and which specific strategies will work best for you.

3. Find out how you are actually coping with your stress on the Stressed-Out Scale. Are you a candidate for burnout, in burnout, or in adrenal fatigue?

After you take the quiz, you'll have the opportunity to talk directly with Dr. Lewis to find out what you can do to reverse the signs of stress.

The consultation is guaranteed to provide you with deeper insight into your state of stress and health. You will be inspired to move forward with additional strategies and tips to reduce your tension, live healthier, and take control of your life.

Get your free quiz at
www.StopStressingMeOut.com/quiz

About the Author

Who is Dr. Lisa Lewis?

Are you a person who feels tired or exhausted all the time? As you age (gracefully, of course), are you feeling more aches and pains, or every month a different part of your body doesn't work like it used to? Are you all work and no play, or all work then pass out as soon as you get home, sit down, or lie down?

Have you been to doctors time and time again complaining that you don't feel well, but they can't figure out what's wrong? Or have they told you to take it easy and slow down because your stress level is making you sick, but no one's taught you how slow down? You have a million things to do, not enough time to do them, and the bills have to get paid. When are you supposed to find time to slow down?

Many of your condition may be stress-related. And there's no pill to treat stress. Through her work as a naturopathic physician and acupuncturist, Dr. Lisa Lewis has treated tons of patients with both acute and chronic diseases, but stress-related disease has become one of her specialties, since she's practiced in and around major metropolitan areas. She has had great success in helping her patients adjust their lifestyles, overcome overwhelm and disease, and live healthier lives. That is why this book was written: with the hope that you can implement some of these strategies and gain the success that Dr. Lewis's patients have received.

Dr. Lewis was dedicated to becoming a doctor at a very early age. She worked for the pharmaceutical industry for many years, but became disillusioned with the healthcare system. She began searching for alternatives to complimentary and conventional medicine, and her curiosity led her to alternative medicine, nutrition, herbal medicine, and dietary supplements to treat and prevent illness. She was immediately struck by the common sense of it all and began to implement these alternative medicine strategies in her own life.

She graduated from Bastyr University with a doctorate in naturopathic medicine, a master in acupuncture, and a certificate in Chinese herbal medicine. These natural medicine principles are the basis for this book, *Stop Stressing Me Out,* and her practice. Dr. Lewis is also the co-author of the e-book *3 Days to Detox: The Step by Step Guide for Busy People to Naturally Lose Weight and Feel Great.*

Dr. Lewis is no stranger to stress, based on her difficult personal life situations, her intense educational pursuits, and her challenging work experiences. She works tirelessly to continue her commitment to being a lifelong learner, but also endeavors to reduce her stress and create balance in her life. She practices the strategies in *Stop Stressing Me Out*: nutrition, acupuncture, meditation, relaxation, exercise, natural remedies and supplements, and adrenal and neurotransmitter testing, and has used them to help heal her life.

Your life and perspective on health will be greatly impacted by *Stop Stressing Me Out*. Here's to relieving stress, overcoming overwhelm and disease, and living healthy the natural way.

Contents

Introduction:
How Much Stress Do You Really Have?...................... 1

Part 1: Why Are You Stressed Out? 7

Chapter 1: The Age of Stress: Today's New Silent Epidemic 9
Learn the science behind how stress truly affects your body.

Chapter 2: What Does Your Stress Feel Like? Mental and Emotional Stress 19
Create an awareness of your mental and emotional stressors, and how they affect your body.

Chapter 3: Your Finances and Personal Management Choices are Stressing You Out 25
Understand your financial and personal stressors, and how they affect your body.

Part 2: 7 Solutions to Overcome Overwhelm & Conquer Disease *Naturally* 31

Chapter 4: Solution # 1: The Joy of Food: Food is Medicine ...33
Discover how food plays an important part in managing and eliminating your stress, including what to eat and stress-free recipes.

Chapter 5: Solution # 2: Nature's Stress Relief: The Healing Power of Vitamins, Mineral, Herbs, Essential Oils, and Water 53
Learn how you can use natural substances such as vitamins, minerals, herbs, supplements, essential oils, and water to reduce your stress, including a formula for stress relief.

Chapter 6: Solution # 3: Acupuncture—The Stress Reliever: No Pain…All Gain 67
Understand the power of acupuncture to help release stress from your body and keep you balanced.

Chapter 7: Solution # 4: Breath of Life—Deep Breathing, Meditation, and Relaxation Strategies 77
Practice deep breathing, meditation, and relaxation techniques with exercises to help melt the stress from your body.

Chapter 8: Solution # 5: Exercise, It Does a Body Good—or Maybe Not? 87
Differentiate whether exercise could help you and why it shouldn't always be recommended when you're too stressed out.

Chapter 9: Solution # 6: Relax, Relate, Relieve: Melt Your Stress Away 97
Connect with the importance that sleep, rest, and fun have on your stress level, and how they can be used to eliminate stress from your body.

Chapter 10: Solution # 7: Naturopathic Medicine: Health Care's Best Kept Secret 107
Taking natural medicine to the next level and understanding how a visit with me as a naturopathic physician and acupuncturist will help you eliminate stress and overcome disease, including case studies.

Introduction

How Much Stress Do You Really Have?

"If I had my way I'd make health catching instead of disease."
~Robert Ingersoll

Health is a normal state. It's when your body is balanced, in a state of homeostasis, and working efficiently. When you're healthy, normal body function is effortless.

When it takes significant effort to maintain body function, that's not normal, yet lately, most people need to apply more and more daily effort to staying healthy, all the while calling their life normal.

Additionally, people misunderstand normal. They believe that health is a state of more, a sort of high. They search for health and expect it to feel like they have superpowers. Normal and healthy is a state of zero, a state of balance, feeling good.

But let's observe normal for a moment. Think back to when you had a toothache -- that throbbing, achy, sharp pain that your mind constantly focused on. Was that normal? No, normal is painless or lack of awareness of your tooth.

And when your tooth was painful, you yearned for normal. You actually appreciated normal when you're tooth was aching, but when you felt well, your mind didn't need to give that tooth any real attention.

Now, let's consider normal as it relates to lab tests. In general, lab test results can fall within the normal range, high or low. But there is also another option - optimal range. Optimal range is still within the normal range, but it's a higher state of normal. This state of optimal is what I consider normal. It's when your body is working at its best state possible. This is the state I reach for when treating patients.

Since healing is also a natural, normal state, you have a higher capacity to heal when you are in an optimal / normal state. Even though stress is inevitable in your life, constant, chronic stress is not normal. Therefore, you must release the stress out of your body and mind, with the goal of being as normal or stress free as possible to maintain optimal health.

> *Thinking back, I remember when I first really started feeling ill, I was 25 years old. I thought it was just a change I was going through, I thought it was temporary. But I didn't realize that stress was the primary cause of my symptoms. After all, who could be stressed at 25?*
>
> *Well, 25 was a big year for me. Not only had I worked really hard most of my life, but I bought my first house that year. I didn't even realize that I had fear and anxiety around making that level of commitment, but my body started telling me with symptoms. I had severe hormonal imbalances, food allergies, digestive problems, and fatigue.*
>
> *One symptom after another showed up, and I never connected them to stress. I wasn't doing anything that was abnormal for me. My life was full of demands and I had been functioning at the same pace for at least the 10 years prior. I was so disconnected that I didn't even know I was stressed. It was my norm.*
>
> *I tried to get answers from so many doctors who wanted to prescribe drugs and surgery, but I was never offered solutions. I was constantly told, there's nothing wrong its just the aging process. My quality of life was decreasing year by year and no one had any answers.*
>
> *Since I was in the medical field and my childhood goal was*

Introduction – How Much Stress Do You Really Have?

*to be a physician, I began exploring my health options and I finally found Naturopathic Medicine. It offered real answers to my problems. It addressed the underlying cause of my symptoms and I decided to go to medical school and study **that** medicine. I became my first patient, and so my journey began.*

After graduating, the stress got worse and the symptoms of severe hormonal imbalances, food allergies, digestive problems, and fatigue also got worse. Real life took over and burnout set in. I finally tested myself and I was in full blown adrenal fatigue. Implementing all the solutions in this book helped me heal myself. So, I turned my own personal growth and healing into a methodology to treat my patients.

No one completely understands the ill effects of stress on your life and how it causes disease more than I do. I have experienced a life full of prolonged, chronic stress, many times self-imposed (athletics, medical school, and personal tragedies). You name it, I've been through it.

This book is a compilation of many of the modalities and treatment therapies I utilized over the years of treating myself and patients for a variety of diseases caused by stress. As a Naturopathic Physician and Acupuncturist, I realized that my patients experience levels of stress that where so high, it compromised their health and quality of life.

Without addressing the stress in their lives directly, many other therapies or treatments they utilized netted mediocre results at best. Once I began to treat their stress, which in many cases was the true cause of their condition, most of their illness, and chronic diseases, began improving and in many cases simply disappeared.

This book is for anyone who is currently experiencing stress in their life or has experienced prolonged periods of chronic stress. If you are suffering from Chronic Diseases such as: Hypertension, Diabetes, Anxiety, Depression, Insomnia (sleep disorders), Weight gain/Obesity, Allergies, Asthma, Migraines, Cardiovascular diseases, digestive problems, this book is for you.

You may have Skin Disorders or Hormonal Imbalances. You may be a woman suffering from disorders, including but not limited to Infertility, PMS, Fibroids, Menstrual Disorders, Hot Flashes. You may be a man suffering from disorders, including but not limited to prostate disease, impotence, premature ejaculation. If you have pain, arthritis, gum diseases, inflammation, auto-immune disorders, etc., treating your stress is essential.

The primary natural solutions detailed in this book include:

Therapeutic Nutrition, Dietary Counseling, Herbal Medicine, Acupuncture and Chinese Herbal Medicine, Detoxification / Cleansing, Aromatherapy, Exercise, Meditation, Counseling (talk therapy), and other Stress Reduction Techniques.

If you follow the strategies detailed in this book you will:

- discover secrets to better cope with your daily stress,
- discover how to interchange stress releasing strategies based on the amount and type of stress you experience, which will ultimately help you get better results,
- learn how to stop stressing out even if you are on a budget and don't want to spend a lot of money,
- discover how to prevent the effects of future stress on your body,
- discover how to use your mental and emotional power to minimize the effect of stress on your body,
- discover how your mental and emotional power can help improve your motivation so you can pursue your life purpose

This book provides an understanding of many treatment modalities and how natural medicine can be used to manage your everyday stress. I encourage you to read this book and implement

Introduction – How Much Stress Do You Really Have?

the solutions provided. You can take your healing journey further than you would otherwise travel if you were simply using standard medicine and chasing symptoms.

> "Give your stress wings and let it fly away."
> - *Terri Guillemets*

Breathe in the energy of life from the top of the head letting it fill all of your body with rejuvenating, vital healing energy. Breathe deeply through the nose and exhale slowly and completely through the mouth. Breathe in, using the diaphragm, pushing the abdomen out, completely filling you lower and upper lungs. Exhale. Now take another deep breath and let's begin!

Part 1

Why Are You Stressed Out?

Chapter 1

The Age of Stress: Today's New Silent Epidemic

"Stress should be a powerful driving force, not an obstacle."
~ Bill Phillips

Stress: Its Nature and Causes

Stress. Everyone's intimately attached to it—some more than others—but let's talk about how stress shows up in *your* life.

Stress is natural, it's an everyday occurrence, and it happens in everyone's life. If you are living in today's society, you have stress, but in today's technology-driven, fast-paced, microwave society, stress is one of your greatest liabilities, especially as it relates to your health and well-being.

Your body is designed to handle stress—to experience stress. Someone said that you should not sweat the small stuff, and by the way it's all small stuff. So, if your mind recognizes any stuff, small or large, the body will react to it.

You are exposed to so many stressors every day in your environment that it's nearly impossible not to have a physical reaction to stress. What you need to learn is how to handle that stress. The goal is reducing the amount of stress in your life and learning how to respond to the stress that is inevitable in your life.

Positive and Negative Stressors

For the most part, *stress* is perceived as a negative word. Just saying or thinking of the word *stress* brings about a negative emotion or feeling. But let's keep in mind is that stress can be both positive and negative. It just really depends on how you view things.

For example, positive stressors can include having fun with friends, getting married, planning a wedding—well, maybe planning the wedding can periodically fall in the negative stressor category. A few more examples of positive stressors are getting a promotion or pay raise, the birth of a baby, and fun activities like riding a roller coaster (as long as you don't fear roller coasters).

You're familiar with negative stressors, which could include financial problems, relationship problems, loss of a family member or friend, problems at work, accidents, injuries, disease, over-committing ourselves, tweens and teenagers, etc. These are emotional stressors.

Stress also have an effect on you physically: exposure to chemicals, disease, accidents, injuries, malnutrition, allergies, pain, too much caffeine, not enough sleep, hormonal disorders, smoking, poor eating habits, too much noise in your life, sedentary lifestyle, addictions that include alcohol, and—yes, ladies—chocolate.

Acute or Chronic Stress

Stressors can also be defined as short-term (acute) or long-term (chronic).

Acute Stress

Acute stress is the reaction to an immediate threat, commonly known as the *fight or flight response*. The threat can be any situation that you experience, even if you only think about it subconsciously. Common acute stressors include:

- Noise (which can trigger a stress response even during sleep)

Chapter 1: The Age of Stress: Today's New Silent Epidemic

- Crowding
- Isolation
- Hunger
- Danger (any kind)
- Infection
- Technology (e.g., TV, video games, cell phones)
- Imagining a threat or remembering a dangerous event

Normally, once the acute stress has passed, the response becomes inactivated and your stress hormones return to normal, a condition called the *relaxation response.*

Chronic Stress

Unfortunately and frequently, however, modern life causes never-ending stressful situations that are not short-term and the urge to act (to fight or to flee) must be suppressed. Stress, then, becomes chronic. Common chronic stressors include:

- Persistent financial worries
- Ongoing highly pressured work or life
- Long-term relationship problems
- Long-term bad lifestyle habits
- Loneliness
- Disease or illness

Long-term chronic stress leads to dis-ease. Common symptoms and diseases caused by stress are listed on the following pages.

Common Symptoms Caused by Stress

Emotional

Absentmindedness
Alternating moods
Aloofness
Anguish
Anger
Annoyance
Anxiety
Apathy
Apprehension
Anti-social behavior
Blaming others
Concentration, lack of
Confidence, lack of
Concerned, overly
Criticism, excessive
Delusions
Dementia
Despondency
Disoriented
Discontent
Discouragement
Dissatisfaction
Doubts
Dreams, nightmares
Drowsiness
Embittered
Failures
Fear, unexplained
Fixed ideas
Frustration
Fussiness
Grief
Hate
Hesitancy, often
Hopelessness, feelings of
Impatience
Impulsiveness
Indecision
Indifference
Intolerance
Interest, lack of
Irritability
Learning, inability
Loneliness
Melancholy
Moodiness
Nervousness
Obsessive-compulsive behavior
Over-sensitivity
Panic
Poise, lack of
Pre-senility, senility
Procrastination
Psychoses
Revengefulness
Restlessness
Ruminative thoughts
Sadness
Self-blaming
Self-centeredness
Self-confidence, lack of
Self-dislike
Self-pity
Self-reproach
Sensitivity
Shyness
Sleeping disorders
Suicidal tendencies
Sulkiness
Talkativeness
Tearfulness
Tension
Terror
Tormented
Uncertainty
Unhappiness
Vexation
Violent behavior
Weariness
Worry

Chapter 1: The Age of Stress: Today's New Silent Epidemic

Physical

Convulsions
Energy, lack of
Exhaustion
Faintness
Headaches
Impotence
Muscle spasms
Neuralgia
Numbness
Over-exercising
Pain, vague
Sex disturbances
Strain
Stuttering
Tension headaches
Vertigo
Weight gaining (non-endocrine)

Common Diseases Caused by Stress

Acne
Aging (premature)
Alcoholism
Allergies
Alzheimer's disease
Angina pectoris
Anorexia nervosa
Arrhythmias
Asthma
Bulimia
Cancer (all forms)
Cerebral vascular accident (stroke)
Colitis (ulcerative, Crohn's disease)
Cushing's disease
Depression (all forms)
Diabetes (certain forms)
Diabetic neuritis
Diabetic retinopathy
Drug/substance addiction
Eczema
Epilepsy
Gum diseases (peridontal)
Hypertension (high blood pressure)
Hypoglycemia (low blood sugar)
Impotence
Infertility
Insomnia
IBS (irritable bowel syndrome)
Glaucoma (open angle)
Menopausal Symptoms
Menstrual disorders
Migraine headaches
Multiple sclerosis
Myocardial infarction (heart attack)
Myasthenia gravis
Narcolepsy
Obesity (non-endocrine)
Psoriasis
Parkinson's disease
Pruritus ani (certain forms)
Schizophrenia
Stuttering
Tinnitus
Trigeminal neurologia
Ulcers, gastric and duodenal
Viral infections (recurrent)

How many times has this happened to you?

You got out of bed late this morning because you kept hitting the snooze button. You just couldn't get to sleep last night—or the three nights before. You rush out of the house, and 15 minutes into your commute you realize you left a file at home that you need for your 9:00 a.m. meeting this morning. It's too late to turn around, so you continue to work.

You drive 10 more minutes and traffic comes to a dead stop. Because you're running late you didn't get a chance to check the traffic. You're already 20 minutes behind schedule, and then there's an accident with no alternate route in sight.

So you sit there for the next 30 min., knowing you're going to be late for your meeting, which you aren't prepared for. You call the office with that familiar "stuck in traffic" story and tell them you'll be there as soon as possible.

How You Are Affected by Stress

Your body maintains a delicate balance (homeostasis) that helps your body function properly and manage stress on a daily basis. When that balance is interrupted symptoms arise. Stressors cause imbalances in your endocrine system (hormones), nervous system (neurotransmitters), and immune system.

This is important because many of the common problems people suffer from today can be associated with stress, but not much is being done about the cause (which is reducing the stress). Most treatment is directed at the symptoms, which quite frankly doesn't work very well. These symptoms wouldn't need to be treated if the cause (stress) was addressed. That's why this book is designed to provide solutions to the stress problem.

Common symptoms of insomnia, fatigue, and anxiousness each affect 40–75 million people in America. If we add menopausal symptoms, mood swings, persistent illness, weight management issues, focus and concentration issues, blood sugar, and digestive disorders, we can literally touch almost everyone in America.

Chapter 1: The Age of Stress: Today's New Silent Epidemic

The Endocrine System and What Are Hormones?

Endocrinology is the study of the body's organs and glands, along with hormone production and activity, and disease states. Endocrine glands include the adrenals, ovaries, testes, pancreas, pituitary, hypothalamus, thyroid, and parathyroid.

Hormones are biochemical messengers used by the endocrine system to communicate with itself and the rest of the body systems. Hormones are involved in many functions, including bone growth and sugar regulation. Hormones can also be involved in disease states such as diabetes and obesity.

The Nervous System and Neurotransmitters

The nervous system is the primary communication system in the body. Neurons (nerve cells) release neurotransmitters, which are chemicals your body uses to relay information and communicate within nervous system.

Chronic stress is the primary contributor to neurotransmitter imbalance. Stress, both emotional and physical, can cause neurons to release large amounts of neurotransmitters to help you cope with each situation.

Acute stress is generally tolerated very well and doesn't cause significant neurotransmitter imbalances. In contrast, chronic or day-in, day-out stress, from things like a busy career, a stressed relationship, or a bacterial or viral infection, will tax the nervous system, and over time deplete your neurotransmitter supplies.

The complete details explaining the interplay between hormones and neurotransmitters is beyond the scope of this book. The basic take-home message is that the behind the scenes the body has mechanisms to manage stress, and when stress is prolonged the balancing act is compromised.

This rest of the chapter will give you a working understanding of the physiology of stress. This is exactly how your body reacts to stress. We will primarily discuss the adrenal gland since its primary function is to manage stress.

The Adrenal Gland

The adrenal glands are two small triangular glands. One gland sits on top of each kidney. There are two distinct parts of the adrenal gland: the cortex and medulla. These parts produce hormones and neurotransmitters.

The cortex produces the hormones cortisol and DHEA, and the medulla produces the neurotransmitters, epinephrine (adrenaline), and norepinephrine (noradrenaline). The adrenal glands are also a secondary production site for sex hormones (testosterone, estrogen, progesterone).

Cortisol is the hormone of stress. It is produced by your adrenals when activated by stress. Cortisol, along with epinephrine (adrenaline), prepares your body for stressful situations by increasing mental alertness, heart rate, metabolism, blood pressure, etc. It is also triggered when you exercise.

Cortisol is a very powerful anti-inflammatory, and releases sugar from the liver and muscles into your blood for instant fuel. It is classified as a fat burner and along with epinephrine helps release fat from the fat cells. However, excess cortisol can cause you to store fat around the midsection.

Stages of Stress Response and Adrenal Fatigue

Early Stage

This is acute stress. Your cortisol, DHEA, epinephrine, and norepinephrine are elevated. This is true flight or fight. Your symptoms in this stage could be overstimulation, anxiety, insomnia, ADHD, and high blood pressure.

Once your stressful situation is over, the cortisol, DHEA, epinephrine, and norepinephrine levels should go back to normal.

Mid-Stage

If stress continues for a prolonged period of time, and your cortisol level remains high, then cortisol becomes an important destructive force that affects practically each cell or organ in your body.

Chapter 1: The Age of Stress: Today's New Silent Epidemic

Eventually, the adrenal glands weaken and start to under-produce cortisol. The DHEA, epinephrine, and norepinephrine may be elevated or low, or fluctuate between low and high during in this stage. Your symptoms may show up as a wired but tired feeling and depression.

The medulla is especially prone to damage from over-stimulation. Also, overproduction of epinephrine can lead to symptoms such as chronic fatigue, irritability, anxiety, panic attacks, tantrums, insomnia, nervous exhaustion or breakdown, inability to relax, pacing, twitching, depression, and feelings of helplessness.

End Stage: Adrenal Exhaustion

Once stress is chronic the adrenal glands are producing very little cortisol. All hormones and neurotransmitters (cortisol, DHEA, epinephrine, and norepinephrine) are depressed. These levels are not high enough for daily function. Symptoms of exhaustion are difficulty dealing with stress, fatigue, cognitive decline, and weight gain.

These symptoms are pretty severe, but unfortunately common in this society, and not often tied to stress and adrenal fatigue. The goals of this chapter are knowledge and awareness. Once you hear and know this information, you will have the power to make the changes in your life necessary to overcome stress and its symptoms.

Lifestyle plays a huge part in how stress affects your body. If you have even a small amount of stress, it is important to take good care of your body or your adrenal glands will fatigue faster. The following are ways your adrenal glands can become exhausted with over-stimulation:

- Caffeinated products (coffee, soda, tea, and chocolate)
- Alcohol (beer, wine, or mixed drinks)
- Drugs (recreational and medications)
- Pesticides, chemicals, and hormones found in our vegetables and meats

- Food preservatives, dyes, synthetic sugars, hydrogenated oils, skin creams, makeup, shampoos, and perfumes
- Poor diet and lifestyle

The details of how to assess and treat the endocrine and nervous systems will be discussed further in Chapter 10 (Solution #7: Naturopathic Medicine).

In the meantime, sit back relax, and begin learning the 7 Solutions to Overcome Overwhelm and Conquer Disease Naturally. While you're reading, try some of the exercises and techniques, and hopefully you can start reducing your stress even before you complete this book.

Chapter 2

What Does Your Stress Feel Like? Mental and Emotional Stress

"You can change the world by changing yourself."
-Author Unknown

This is one of my favorite quotes because it so exemplifies what humankind knows in their hearts to be true. If you truly want things to change in your life, whether in your home, your work, your town, your state, or your country, looking to others to make the change for you is futile. You have to be the change you want to see.

Mental and Emotional Stress

When you change how you see yourself and how you see others, things always look little brighter. No matter what the situation, it will always appear better with a positive outlook. You know people like this. They always have a smile on their face and a positive outlook on every situation. They see the beauty and grace in everything.

Conversely, no matter how great life appears to be through the eyes of others, if people have a negative outlook, attitude, or prospective, things will always appear dimmer. These people never seem to be truly happy, but on the outside appear to have everything others dreams of.

Stress affects your mental, emotional, and physical states. Your mind doesn't know the difference between an actual experience and the thought of the experience. For example, the body can react to a physical trauma in the same way that it reacts to simply thinking about the trauma.

Knowing that alone can be an eye-opening experience. Could you imagine how the body reacts to a gory scene from a horror movie, constantly being yelled at, and bullied, or how the mind perceives the violence of video games?

Therefore, it's important to remember that your thoughts and words have power. When you experience trauma, the energy and experience are held in your body. The emotion and physical experience can be experienced over and over again.

Most people have heard the phrase *your words and your thoughts have power*. Well, truly understanding that what you say and think can be translated to actual physical effects in your body is very powerful indeed. What you say can and does actually come true.

Experiencing negative situations, having negative thoughts, and existing in negative circumstances can have a detrimental effect on your health. They are defined as stress, and stress has been associated with many diseases and illnesses.

Stop and think for a minute. Have you ever been in pain? I want you to try a brief exercise I've tried many times. The next time you find yourself in pain—a headache, stomach ache, whatever pain sensation it may be—stop and take yourself to a pleasant place. Try to remove yourself mentally from the pain.

Instead of focusing on how much it hurts, focus on something else—an object or a pleasant memory. Within a few seconds you will find that your pain level has decreased.

This is just one example of the power of the mind. You can see just how powerful it is. You can experience how simply thinking of and taking yourself to a better place—thinking positively or pleasantly—can instantaneously make your world better. If you can stand in that space, your world will be better.

Chapter 2: What Does Your Stress Feel Like? Mental and Emotional Stress

What Does Your Stress Feel Like?

If you're reading this book, you're probably old enough to have experienced emotional challenges or trauma. But how can you connect those emotions to a physical condition? The mind-body connection is not commonly taught in this society.

Emotional stress can stay with you for much longer than you can imagine. Without releasing the emotion and removing the stress, a physical challenge is sure to follow.

Some people never release emotional stress. They take their anger, their fear, their frustration, and their sadness with them everywhere they go, every day of their life. This is the very definition of chronic stress.

In Chapter 1 (Stress 101), diseases and symptoms associated with stress were listed, and many of you were probably surprised. But if you really sit back and think—really think—about when you began to feel or experience a disease, condition, or symptom, you may be able to relate it back to an emotion or traumatic experience in your life.

Maybe there are one or two experiences you never let go of, and that emotion or feeling was never released. But it had to go somewhere. So again, it finds itself in an area of our body that is susceptible, weak, or previously injured, and the disease process continues.

Think positive thoughts, live a more positive life, and see how your physical body responds. Then see how the world around you reacts to that positivity. Part 2 of this book will discuss techniques and strategies for releasing emotional and mental stress.

Does this sound like you?

Your doctor asks you, "On a scale of one to ten, with one being no stress and ten the most stress you ever had, what would you say your stress level is regularly?"

You answer, "About two to three out of ten. I don't really have much stress."

Your doctor says, "Okay, let's examine that closer. Describe a normal day for you."

You respond, "I get out of bed by 5:15 a.m., I'm showered and dressed by 6:15 a.m., I prepare breakfast for the family, leave the house around 7 a.m., commute 45 minutes to one hour to work, work all day sometimes without a lunch and meetings straight through until the end of the day.

I leave work to commute home at about 6:00 p.m., I arrive home at approximately 7:00 p.m., I cook dinner, I spend an hour or two with my husband and family, and I fall asleep between 11:30 p.m. and 12:00 a.m. Then I get up and do the same thing all over again, five days a week.

My weekends are filled with running the errands that I can't run during the week, such as grocery shopping, taking the kids to their events, cleaning the house, any additional shopping, planning meals for the week, preparing Sunday dinner, exercising, spending some time with friends and family, and a bit of relaxation.

I'm exhausted all the time and don't have any time for myself. I feel like every minute of every day is planned and I have no breathing room. This is my schedule every week of every month except when I go on vacation."

If this sounds like you or if your schedule is even worse than this, I have news for you: Your stress level is not two to three out of ten. It is much, much higher. It may appear to be two to three because you've gotten used to it; it's your daily routine, it's your life. But just because you're used to it doesn't mean your body doesn't respond to the same way it would if this was your schedule once in a blue moon.

Keeping a schedule like this will lead to chronic stress. That's why the woman in this example says she's exhausted. Her body just can't keep up with her schedule. Her pace is unrealistic and it will

Chapter 2: What Does Your Stress Feel Like? Mental and Emotional Stress

catch up to her sooner or later. But if this is you, you might not feel fatigue alone. It could show up as any hosts of diseases.

For example, if your lungs are weak, it may show up as asthma or allergies. If your digestion is weak, it could show up as IBS (irritable bowel syndrome), food allergies, headaches, nausea, indigestion, etc. If your muscles are weak, it could show up as muscle cramps, pain, tightness, weakness, etc. Get the picture? Stress can hit you where ever it can, *and it will!*

Chapter 3:

Your Finances and Personal Management Choices are Stressing You Out

"The greatest wealth is health."
~ Virgil

Nobody knows better than I the challenges that limited finances can have on your stress level.

Growing up in a lower-middle-class family, it was not really understood that money was an issue. For the most part, I had all the things that I needed and wanted. But as it became time for me to take care of myself, financial stress became an issue.

I had to work many jobs and long hours while attending college. I primarily had loans and scholarships to pay for school, but any incidentals that were required were hard to come by. The difficulties of passing my classes as a premed student, working, and having a little fun took a significant toll on me.

The same situation occurred with medical school, except for one caveat: Before medical school I had a great job and lots of money, which I had to give up to go back to school. The stress of remembering being a broke college student stayed with me and was compounded by significant lifestyle change from flourishing professional to unemployed medical student.

Additionally, after graduating, starting my own business from scratch, and building it up to see the recession take a hatchet to it, was very difficult. To see all the work for your career, your home, and your possessions all in jeopardy, due to significant financial challenges is stress indeed.

Along with the stress, my health deteriorated, as well as my career and my financial nest egg. With medical bills and all other bills mounting, it was very difficult to pull myself up by my bootstraps.

You see, stress could have been the cause or the results of my health problems. I still don't know which came first, the chicken or the egg, but I know financial stress definitely contributed to my health problems.

Stress and Your Finances

What are you going through financially? Is your life made more stressful by financial challenges? This question is for people with high incomes as well as low, since the adage tends to be true: The more money you make, the more money you spend.

Financial stress is a significant stressor in many people's lives, and the topic is going to be addressed in this chapter. Although it can be a sensitive topic, the best way to address it is head on.

Financial stress and money management go hand in hand. As mentioned in the previous chapter, emotions and the mind-body connection isn't readily discussed in this society. Well, money management is another topic that isn't openly discussed. If more people were taught how to manage money, financial matters would not be a significant stressor in this society.

You thought this book was supposed to be a stress-management book, not a finance book. Well, you are 100 percent correct. This book was written to provide solutions for stress reduction, but since financial stress is so high on the list of stressors in today's society, a brief discussion on financial stress would be helpful. Let's begin.

Everyone starts off with a number, which can be called

Chapter 3: Your Finances and Personal Management Choices are Stressing You Out

income. They also have financial responsibilities and a lifestyle that is essential to maintain, which can be called expenses. If their expenses are less than their income, their stress is probably low to normal. If, however, the opposite is true and the expenses equal or exceed their income, their stress is probably high.

You can only shift this scenario in a few ways. To reduce stress you can increase your income, reduce your expenses, or both. I know this sounds simplistic, but it's true.

Financial management and stress management basics really boil down to simple arithmetic. In order to reduce financial stress it's essential to understand money management, create and follow a budget, and practice a certain level of financial discipline. These are the essential basics.

Everyone's situation changes due to life circumstances, but understanding which equation describes your current or past financial situation will usually determine if you suffer from financial stress.

Poverty Consciousness

"The greatest weapon against stress is our ability to choose one thought over another."
~ *William James*

Poverty is not just the state of physical being or lack of money, but also a state of mind—something called poverty consciousness or lack mentality. Knowing that they don't have something today affects people for the moment. But thinking they will never have anything, and living life without the expectation of change, growth, or hope, can keep the physical body in a perpetual state of stress.

This is why it's so important to always believe that something better or different is possible. The cells in your body don't know the difference between poverty or riches, they only respond to the negative or positive experience. So, think positively and let your cells respond to the hope that your poverty state will change.

The poverty mindset does not necessarily have to do with being poor. It has to do with the overall concept of possibilities in one's life. It also has to do with not creating the resources necessary to maintain one's lifestyle. Nevertheless, and especially in this economy, financial challenges have a significant affect on your health and well-being.

It's common for people to think they don't have stress in many other areas of their life, and it's equally difficult for them to connect with financial stress. So their finances, or lack thereof, can't be making them sick, right? Please know that if finances are one of the leading factors in divorce and myriad other problems, they could also be a significant contributing factor to your health.

Does this mean that because you're financially strapped you'll never be healthy? Absolutely not, it just means beware! Of all the contributing factors that can cause your health to decline, and very quickly, finances are at the top of the list.

Simply knowing this can help reduce the effect that financial problems can have on your health. With knowledge comes power. You can counteract the effects of stress, but you first have to know that you are experiencing stress.

Money, Money, Money

Conversely, others show what appears to be the opposite of poverty consciousness. Their attachment to money shows up differently. These are the people who hoard money or simply focus too much attention on acquiring it.

At first glance, it would appear that this imbalance couldn't produce stress—because, after all, if a person has money what is there to stress about, right? Wrong.

Oftentimes the activities leading up to acquiring money and the activities required to maintain money, also lead to high stress. Just think of the jobs that are high-reward, high-income, but very high-stress (for example, stock brokers, management consultants who travel four or five days a week, high-end sales jobs, physicians, lawyers, entrepreneurs, etc.).

Chapter 3: Your Finances and Personal Management Choices are Stressing You Out

Remember that this is simply another viewpoint. The effects of stress are pervasive. Just because people are used to a certain level of stress doesn't mean it affects them any less. All stress eventually takes a toll on your health. Awareness and changing habits today can help tons for the future.

Organization and Time Management Stress

The saying goes "the early bird catches the worm." But, you can be sure that the early bird had a plan. It woke up early with a purpose. For instance, it's very probable that the bird knew when to wake up, where the worms hang out, what time the worms arrive, and how many worms it could catch in a certain amount of time. Yup, that bird had a plan; otherwise, the bird and its family may go hungry.

The more you think ahead about how to manage activities or control your time, the less stress you will experience. One of the easiest ways to manage your time is to make a to-do list and prioritize your demands daily. Many people make lists without priorities, and others make lists and then never use them.

It's always best to create a prioritized plan with specific time scheduled for each activity. Managing your time and adjusting your schedule to ensure you focus on or complete the issues/projects that are most important to you helps to reduce and control your stress.

How would you like more time in your day to practice some of the stress-reduction solutions and relaxation techniques you're going to learn in Part 2 of this book? A large part of your day is usually eaten up by activities that are dropped into your lap or thrust upon you without your permission. Controlling your time and taking charge of your time will really free up valuable energy you can use to spend fulfilling your goals instead of putting out fires.

No More Drama: Remove Your Stress

Are you the kind of person who says "of course" or "sure" without even thinking first, and then later you feel a knot in your

29

stomach when someone—anyone—asks you to take on yet another project? Do you take on more projects even though you know you already have more responsibilities than you can handle? This section is definitely for you. It's time to set some limits for your self and practice self-care.

No more promising more than you can achieve comfortably. Determine, on your own time and alone if possible, what you can realistically do. This means what you can do without burning yourself out. Then, like the war on drugs slogan, "just say no"—though you can say it politely.

Also, begin to take stock in the things that are creating stress in your life. One by one, begin to assess these situations, people, or things that contribute to your stress and adjust how you interact with them. Do you need the drama? The answer is no!

You can't always just toss a stressor out of the window, but you can change how you show up and deal with it. As discussed in the previous chapter, you can change the world by changing yourself. So remember: Some stress you create can be released, and other stress can be adjusted.

Part 2:

7 Solutions to Overcome Overwhelm & Conquer Disease *Naturally*

Chapter 4

Solution # 1
The Joy of Food: Food is Medicine

"Let medicine be your food and food be your medicine."
~ *Hippocrates*

Can you live without food? Is food a significant part of your life and daily routine? That's why I think the #1 solution to release stress in this society is nutrition. Let's tackle it head on, but gently, or course. Food is a very sensitive subject, and my goal is to help you find the joy and the benefit in food, because you can have both.

Let's get the "stats and stuff" out of the way so we can get to the important stuff: good, healthy food. Unfortunately, the Standard American Diet is frighteningly poor. The typical American eats for convenience, comfort, and taste rather than for fueling the body. The purpose of food is to keep you alive and keep your body mechanisms running efficiently, not simply for taste.

Am I implying that food shouldn't taste good? Absolutely not. Your food should taste great, but taste can't be the only factor to consider when choosing what to eat. It's important to understand how food is viewed in the Western culture and why maintaining a healthy diet is so difficult in today's society.

In many parts of the world, outside of the Western culture, food is medicine. Most cultures eat to live, but the thought process in the Western culture is not to eat to live; it is to live to eat. It's based on taste, which really means how sweet or amazingly pleasing to the palate food is.

Stop Stressing Me Out

Western food labels listing food nutrients are based on viewing the body as machine or laboratory. Food is primarily analyzed and understood based on its parts or constituents. You see it every day: labels listing how much carbohydrate, fat, or protein is contained in food, and very little information about the vitamin and mineral content of food.

Conversely, many outside cultures understand food from the perspective of its behavior once food enters the body. Some foods increase your metabolism, some foods slow you down; some foods generate warmth in the body, some generate cool in the body; some foods are moistening, and some drying.

So how is this information applied? The energetic temperature is based on how food affects you internally, after it's eaten. Energetically warm foods stimulate your digestion and cool foods slow you down. For example, cucumbers, tomatoes, watermelon, and tropical foods are cooling foods, while peppers, lamb, and garlic are warming foods. These foods aren't hot or cold in external temperature; they act in a hot or cold way inside the body.

There are other factors to consider as well. The flavor of food (sweet, pungent, salty, sour, and bitter) can also provide information regarding the action it has on particular organ or system within the body. For example, salty foods affect the kidneys, and sweet food affects the digestive system. If you have an imbalance in an organ, eating foods of a certain flavor can be beneficial. Also, eating foods of a certain flavor too often can create imbalance.

Your diet should also adjust naturally to season and weather changes. You need more warming foods in winter and more cooling foods in summer. In dry climates you need more moistening foods, and in damp climates more drying foods. Moistening food provide lubrication when tissues are too dry, and drying foods pull moisture out of tissues when they are too moist.

For example, dry skin, hair, and constipation need moisture, and oily skin, lung mucous, diarrhea and excess perspiration need drying. Drying foods are arugula, Brussels sprouts, black beans, aduki beans, pumpkin seeds, and trout. Moistening foods are oils, honey, watermelon, spinach, walnuts, beets, cauliflower, salmon, quinoa pears, peaches, and bananas.

Unfortunately our Standard American Diet is overly dependent on wheat, dairy, sugar, meat, and fat, which are dampening foods. Damp foods combined with a sedentary lifestyle put more stress on the body and promote obesity. These damp foods should be offset with the drying foods listed above to reduce their negative affects on the body.

A more appropriate diet would include several more native grains such as rye, barley, and oats, considerably less sugar and dairy (rice, almond, and coconut milk are great dairy substitutes), a wide range of vegetables and fruits, a little fish and meat (less beef and more turkey), and the creative use of a wide variety of edible leafy greens and seeds.

Stress and Nutrition

So what does all this food energetics stuff have to do with stress? Poor dietary habits can contribute to adrenal and neurotransmitter imbalances, especially if a poor diet is combined with high stress.

Here's one example: The production of neurotransmitters depends on adequate levels of amino acid. Since amino acids are the building block of protein, diets low in protein may limit the supplies of these amino acids. Limited protein leads to decreased neurotransmitter levels.

Other dietary factors can also contribute to imbalances. For example, high glycemic (sugar) foods, when eaten in excess, may cause neurotransmitter deficiencies by increasing the release of neurotransmitters.

Another dietary influence concerns appropriate fat intake. Your brain cell membranes are composed primarily of lipids, or fats. Omega-3 fatty acids stabilize these membranes and are required for proper brain cell function. Diets low in these fatty acids can compromise the integrity of the brain cells and lead to faulty neurotransmission. These important dietary fats can be obtained by eating foods rich in omega-3 fatty acids like nuts, seeds, and fish.

Is the point becoming clearer? These examples are primarily based on just the nervous and adrenal systems. The information could go on and on with examples of how nutrients, minerals, and vitamins affect each organ of your body. (That's another book for another day!) You get the point: Food is essential.

Food is really important for the body's internal function, and the fact that it tastes good is secondary. After all, if the body needs food to survive, the taste buds need to make food appetizing or everyone would starve. So, they work together to make sure the species thrives, but being healthy is up to each person individually.

Emotional Eating

Are you the type of person who unconsciously grabs for food when you feel sad, hurt, angry, afraid, or just plain bored? Are you influenced to eat certain foods based on television ads? Does eating just make you feel better, even if it's momentary? If so, you are an emotional eater and you are not alone. That's why it's so important to be conscious of what you eat. If you don't understand what you are craving and why, stress and emotional eating can lead to a very unhealthy lifestyle.

The effect that chronic, uncontrollable stress has on the body and mind gets deeper. Stress not only biases the body to produce more fats, it also begins to influence the type of food you eat, especially through your emotions. Thus, during increased stress people eat more fats than at other times. They tend to increase their fat consumption by as much as 30 percent. Also, a high-fat diet increases the body's production of stress hormones, which also causes weight gain. It's like a viscous cycle.

Look for more on this topic in Chapter 8 (Solution #5: Exercise, It Does the Body Good—or Maybe Not?).

Caffeine Addiction, Sugar Addiction and Stress

Two of America's greatest hidden addictions are caffeine and sugar. Do you have difficulty seeing straight before you have your morning coffee? If so, you may be addicted. Do you crave sugar,

Chapter 4: Solution # 1: The Joy of Food: Food is Medicine

have to eat sweets snacks to stay alert in the afternoon, or find it almost impossible to even think about removing soda, juice, and sugary foods from your diet? If so, you may be addicted to sugar.

It's not your fault. In this fast-paced society it's not difficult to become addicted to sugar or caffeine. Many people need these stimulants to simply keep up with their stressful schedules. Unfortunately, you have a double-edged sword: You need stimulants to keep up with your stressful lifestyle, and the stimulants put even more stress on your body. What a toll this takes on the adrenals.

Part of the addiction is the process. Think of the ritual of drinking coffee. How effective are those coffee television ads showing the pot brewing, with sound effects, and the sleepy household members smelling the aroma and wandering into the kitchen, dressed in pajamas and a comfortable robe, to have their first cup? They make it so enticing.

You can actually cut down your caffeine intake dramatically by slowly reducing the amount you drink daily until you reach a half-cup in the morning and a half-cup in the early afternoon (or even less). Or you can learn to enjoy indulging in a cup of caffeine-free herbal tea. Enjoy the aroma, enjoy the taste, enjoy the ritual of making it, and replace the coffee experience with herbal tea.

Remember that coffee isn't the only source of caffeine. Black teas (such as Lipton) and chocolate also contribute to over-stimulation from caffeine. Another huge source of caffeine is soda. Americans consume a huge amount of soda pop every year, most of which contain caffeine, and all of which either contain unhealthy amounts of sugar, dangerous sugar-replacement products, and/or chemicals.

If sugar isn't listed directly on the ingredients of the package, it's probably disguised as high-fructose corn syrup, which in many respects is worse for the body than sugar. Sugars are also disguised in your diet as bread, white-colored grains, and starchy vegetables. So you say, "I'm not addicted to sugar. My weakness is bread." Bread is a sugar addiction and, from the body's perspective, sugar is sugar. It takes whatever source it can get to feed its addiction.

Caffeine and sugar are associated with stress and anxiety. They cause nervousness, irritation, and heart palpitations. But avoiding other foods and substances are essential for reducing stress, including:

- Salt, which has been associated with heart diseases.
- Cigarettes, which cause tension, irritability, and sleeplessness and have been linked to cancer and heart disease.
- Alcohol, which depletes B vitamins, which are necessary to balance the nervous system.

That's some of the bad news. The good news is that you have me to help guide you through the maze of misinformation. Earlier in the chapter I said my goal was to help you find the joy and the benefit in food, because food can taste good and be good for you. So, let's begin.

Guidelines for Good Food, Good Health, and Stress Reduction

Life and food are about moderation. If you do the right thing most of the time, your health will provide a buffer that allows you to indulge once in a while. Being diligent and seeking the healthy options can be a journey.

Finding substitute ingredients and new recipes can be a bit time-consuming at first, but in the end it's so worth it. And after you've been working so hard at doing the "right" thing, taking a little guilt-free time to indulge feels so good.

Here are general guidelines to help you reduce your food stress and eat healthy:

- Eat a plant-based, predominantly vegetarian diet.
- All produce should be fresh and organic when possible.
- All canned, frozen, and prepackaged foods should be avoided as much as possible.
- Reduce fat intake to 15–20 percent of total calories. Choose

Chapter 4: Solution # 1: The Joy of Food: Food is Medicine

health-promoting fats (essential fatty acids), and avoid saturated and hydrogenated (trans) fats.

- Eat adequate protein (0.8 g per kg of body weight daily) from lean sources such as wild fish, organic poultry and eggs, legumes, low-fat non-fermented dairy products, nuts, and seeds.
- Eat adequate vegetables, fruits, and whole grains, which contain invaluable micronutrients, antioxidants, and fiber.
- Eat at least 30 grams of fiber per day.
- At least half of all vegetables should be eaten raw. The other half should be lightly steamed or baked.
- Eliminate foods with refined sugar and carbohydrates, processed foods, alcohol and caffeine.
- Reduce exposure to pesticides and herbicides by buying organic.
- Fresh food is preferable to frozen food, and frozen food is preferable to canned food.
- Eliminate foods with artificial additives, colors, dyes, preservatives, flavor enhancers, and smoked food and preservatives.
- Identify and eliminate food allergies, intolerances, and sensitivities.
- Determine your caloric needs to achieve or maintain your ideal body weight.
- Avoid soda, artificial drinks and beverages, and stimulant beverages such as coffee and black tea.
- Avoid high sugars, especially refined sugars, high-fructose corn syrup, and artificial sweeteners.
- Avoid all refined, polished grains, flours, and their products.

- All oils should be kept to a minimum, but when used should be cold pressed and refined, and kept refrigerated.
- Salt intake should be low (use naturally processed sea salt or natural tamari) and potassium intake high.
- No deep-frying of any food.
- Avoid white foods.
- Never eat starchy carbohydrates (breads, pastas) by themselves.
- Do not eat foods you crave.
- Avoid foods you are addicted to.
- Avoid foods that make you feel worse, cloud your thinking, or pull you down in any way.
- Never skip breakfast.
- Avoid fruit in the morning (alone). Try to combine fruit with a protein or healthy fat source.
- Chew your food well.

Food Specifics

Whole-Grain Cereals
- Choose brown rice, millet, wheat, rye, barley, oats (oatmeal and oat bran), corn, buckwheat.
- Whole grains are better than flour, which is more difficult to digest, so sprouted breads are preferable.

Vegetables
- Cooking methods include lightly steaming, baking, or sautéing with minimal amounts of sesame or olive oil.
- Fresh vegetable juices and sprouts are both good to include

- but choose homemade juice and make sure you're drinking the whole vegetable. Avoid extracted juices.
- Include large amounts of leafy vegetables, cruciferous vegetables from the cabbage family (cabbage, cauliflower, broccoli, Brussels sprouts, kohlrabi, kale, mustard greens, lettuce, beet greens, chard, collard, bok choy, endive, etc.) and garlic (one to four cloves) daily.
- Include a fair amount of sea vegetables (wakame, nori, kelp, kombu, dulse).
- Keep the nightshade vegetable family to a minimum (tomatoes, eggplant, potatoes, peppers).

Legumes/Beans

- Cook well to increase digestion.
- Choose adzuki beans, mung beans, black-eyed peas, kidney beans, navy beans, red beans, peas, lentils, garbanzo beans, and pinto beans (no peanuts).
- Combine legumes with grains.

Fruits

- Choose fresh, raw, or dried (unsulphered), with dried being best consumed in cooler seasons.
- Preferably choose fruits in season and native to your area and/or climatic zone.

Seeds and Nuts

- The best way to eat seeds is sprouted (alfalfa, radish, sunflower, etc.).
- In small amounts nuts can be enjoyed as snacks (almonds, walnuts, hazel nuts, pecans are best).

- Raw nuts are best soaked overnight before eaten, and stored refrigerated or frozen.

Fish, Poultry, and Dairy

- Eat two to three small servings of white-fleshed (scaled) fish, preferably cold-water species (cod, haddock, sardines, herring, salmon, trout) or white meat poultry, organically and naturally raised (without antibiotics or hormones) and skinned.
- Poaching, steaming, broiling, or in soup, is best.
- Dairy should be avoided in most people. If you can tolerate dairy and are not sensitive to it, organic, hormone-free dairy should consumed.
- Small portions of the harder, non-colored cheeses can be added to the diet, if you are not sensitive to dairy.

Beverages

- Avoid ice-cold beverages. Preferably drink room temperature, or hot/warm teas.
- Drink water when thirsty, but not before or after meals (allow 30–60 minutes).
- Fruit juices should be avoided, but may be consumed in summer in moderation and diluted up to 50 percent with water.
- Recommended daily beverages may include non-caffeinated herbal teas. Also rice, almond, coconut and hemp milk may be included.

Soups

- An excellent addition to daily meals.
- Should include a variety of vegetables, while seaweed is recommended to highlight flavor (preferably wakame, kelp, or dulse).

Simple, Healthy, Stress-Free Recipes

Pumpkin and Chestnut soup
Serves 6

Ingredients:
2 onions
3 tablespoons olive oil
1 medium pumpkin or squash
2 pints vegetable stock
1 cup dried chestnuts, soaked
2 cloves garlic
1 bay leaf
1 teaspoon rosemary
Splash of cider vinegar
Parsley to garnish
Pinch paprika

Method:
Presoak the chestnuts overnight or use fresh chestnuts if available. Chop the onions roughly and fry in the olive oil until softened. Chop the pumpkin, removing the skin and seeds, and sweat with the onions, turning occasionally until it starts to soften.

Add the vegetable stock, chestnuts, crushed garlic, bay leaf and rosemary. Simmer for 40 minutes, remove the bay leaf and puree adding a splash of cider vinegar and a good twist of freshly ground black pepper. Serve garnished with parsley and a sprinkle of paprika.

10 minutes preparation/50 minutes cooking.

Dr. Lewis' Raw Greens Recipe

Serves 5-7

Ingredients:
1 bunch kale or collard greens, stems removed

Marinade:
1/4 cup olive oil and flaxseed oil mixed
1 lemon or lime, juiced
1 Tbls chopped ginger, unpeeled
1/2 onion, cut into crescents
4 cloves of garlic, finely chopped
1/3 cup tamari (wheat free soy sauce)
1 Tbls maple syrup or raw honey
1 Tbls Chinese five spice powder
1/2 tsp cayenne or 1 jalapeno, chopped

Method:

Place collard leaves one on top of the other, next fold them in half. Roll the whole bunch into a tight roll. Starting at one end of the roll, cut the collard greens into very thin slivers and transfer to a large bowl.

Mix together the oil, lemon juice, and the tamari for the marinade. Pour the marinade over the greens and add the other ingredients. Toss well until all the ribbons are well coated. Cover the greens and marinate in the refrigerator minimum of an hour up to overnight (your preference).

This dish will keep for 2-3 days in the refrigerator.
Enjoy!

Chapter 4: Solution # 1: The Joy of Food: Food is Medicine

Salmon Baked In Foil
Serves 1
Preheat oven to 425 degrees F or 200 degrees C.

Ingredients:
4-6 oz salmon
1 -1½ cup fresh spinach
1 tsp grainy mustard or (sugar free dijon mustard)
Sprinkle of sea salt and pepper.

Method:
   Place spinach onto foil square, set fish on top, sprinkle with salt and pepper and smear with grainy mustard. Seal foil tightly and place onto tray. Put into preheated oven. Bake approximately 8 minutes.
   Serve with cabbage and onion.

Curried Vegetables
Serves 1

Ingredients:
½ cup green beans, cut into pieces
½ cup cauliflower, cut into pieces
½ cup eggplant, cut into pieces
½ cup cucumber, cut into pieces
1 clove diced garlic
1 tsp   curry powder
1 tbsp safflower oil
½ cup water

Method:
   Heat oil in saucepan and fry garlic until transparent. Add curry powder and stir through. Add vegetables and ½ cup water. Cook briefly - approximately 5-10 minutes and serve.
   Don't overcook!

Stop Stressing Me Out

Ratatouille
Serves 2

Ingredients:
½ cup   green pepper chopped
½ cup   celery chopped
1 cup   zucchini chopped
1 clove garlic chopped
¼ cup   onion chopped
1 tbsp   parsley chopped
½ cup   tomato chopped
1 tbsp   safflower oil
Sprinkle of dried basil
1 bay leaf (optional)

Method:
   Heat oil in saucepan and fry onion until transparent. Add all the vegetables and spices, close lid firmly on saucepan and simmer over a very low flame. Gradually it will cook to a stew of vegetables. Stir occasionally.
   Serve with any meat or fish or by itself

Dr. Lisa Lewis' Stop Stressing Protein Shakes
Method:
Blend together:

- 2 cups plain almond milk, rice milk or coconut milk (not sweetened vanilla or chocolate flavors, etc.)
- 1 scoop (equivalent to 15 to 20 grams) of protein powder. A non-dairy powder is best (pea, rice, hemp, etc.), measured according to package directions
- 1 cup blueberries or 1 medium banana
- 1 Tbls flaxseed oil or essential oil blend

Chapter 4: Solution # 1: The Joy of Food: Food is Medicine

Further Options

- Add 1 heaping Tbls fiber supplement to the above recipe.
- For extra calories and thickness, add 1-2 Tablespoons nut butter to the above recipe.
- For a "green shake", add powdered spirulina or liquid chlorophyll. Or if you have a powerful blending machine, like a VitaMix, you can add vegetables like Kale, Spinach, Collards, Celery, etc.
- Add 2-3 ice cubes along with cold or frozen fruit and liquid if you want a frosty blend.
- Add 1 cup low fat non-dairy yogurt in place of one cup of liquid for a thicker shake.
- In lieu of blueberries or banana, use 1 cup fresh fruit of your choice, preferably organic, in-season and locally grown.
- You can combine all the ingredients in the blender (except the protein powder and the liquids) ahead of time and refrigerate until you are ready to blend.

There are as many variations to these shakes and smoothies as there are fruit and vegetable options. If you start your day off with this as a meal replacement, it will instantly provide you with more energy and a whole host of vitamins and minerals in the morning. The added bonus is that you get a tasty, low calorie, healthy and balanced breakfast.

But before we end our nutrition exploration, a brief discussion on water and its importance in reducing stress and maintaining health is warranted.

Hydration

"Water is life's matter and matrix, mother and medium. There is no life without water."
~ *Albert Szent-Gyorgyi*

Water is one of the most important substances on the planet. So, it should come as no surprise that water is also one of the most important substances for your body. Water is the main component of the body. It's said that the body is made up of anywhere from 65 to 75 percent water; therefore, it's essential to drink and replenish your body with significant amounts of water every day.

Water content varies depending on your body part:

- Brain consists of 90 percent water.
- Muscle consists of 75 percent water.
- Blood consists of 83 percent water.
- Bone consists of 22 percent of water.

Water bathes your cells, enabling them to function appropriately. Common functions of water are as follows. Water:

- Transports nutrients and oxygen into cells.
- Detoxifies the body.
- Moisturizes the air in lungs.
- Helps with metabolism.
- Helps our organs to absorb nutrients.
- Regulates body temperature.
- Protects our vital organs.
- Protects and moisturizes our joints.

Water has so many amazing benefits for your health and well-being. A few of these benefits are listed here. Water helps you:

Chapter 4: Solution # 1: The Joy of Food: Food is Medicine

1. **Lose weight.** Water flushes out the by-products of fat breakdown. Drinking water also reduces hunger and acts as an effective appetite suppressant. Did you know water has zero calories?

2. **Look younger with healthier skin.** Water helps replenish your skin tissues, moisturizes your skin, and increases your skin elasticity.

3. **Digest and aids with constipation.** Drinking water raises your metabolism because it helps with digestion. Fiber and water work together to help you have daily bowel movements.

4. **Reduce the risk of cancer:** Some studies show that drinking a healthy amount of water may reduce the risks of bladder cancer and colon cancer.

5. **Relieve fatigue.** Water helps you flush out toxins and waste products from your body. If your body lacks water, your organs have to work harder to do their jobs. Your organs will be exhausted and so will you.

6. **Be in a good mood.** Your body feels very good, and that's why you feel happy.

7. **Exercise better.** Drinking water regulates your body temperature. That means you'll feel more energetic when doing exercises. Water also helps to fuel your muscle.

8. **Be less likely to get sick and helps you feel healthy.** Drinking plenty of water helps boost your immune system.

9. **Have better productivity at work.** Your brain is mostly made up of water. Thus drinking water helps you think better, be more alert, and be more concentrated.

10. **Have a natural remedy for headache:** Water helps to relieve headache and back pains due to dehydration.

11. **Have less cramps and sprains:** Proper hydration helps keep your joints and muscles lubricated, so you'll less likely get cramps and sprains.

Dehydration is a huge, practically unrecognized problem in this society. So, how do you know that you're dehydrated and need more water? Here are some of the symptoms that you need more water:

- **Dark urine (dark yellow or orange in color).** Your urine should be pale yellow to clear when you have sufficient water intake. Dark color or a strong smell indicates that you need to drink more water.

- **Dry skin.** Skin is the largest body organ and requires its share of water.

- **Thirst.** Thirst is the most obvious sign that you're already dehydrated. It is always a good practice to drink more water when you are not thirsty; don't wait until you're thirsty.

- **Thirst/hunger reflex.** Most people mistake hunger for the indication to eat more, whereas in fact you may be dehydrated. So before you have your meal, grab a glass of water.

- **Fatigue.** Water is a source of energy and gives you a boost in energy.

As was mentioned earlier, dehydration can have harmful effects on your body. It is important to stay well hydrated. Here are some of the harmful effects of dehydration:

- Tiredness
- Migraines
- Constipation

- Irregular blood pressure
- Kidney problems
- 20 percent dehydrated—risk of death
- Dry skin
- Muscle cramps

Since not drinking enough water puts significant stress on the body, the question is: How much water should you drink a day to avoid dehydration? There's a simple approach of drinking eight glasses of water a day. Is that sufficient?

Here's a more specific approach. Each day your body requires over two quarts (64 ounces) of water in addition to diet in order to function optimally. Heavier people need more water—at least one-third of your body weight in ounces. For example, a 210-pound person needs 70 ounces of water daily.

Caffeine and sugars add to your body's dehydration needs, so add another 8 ounces of water for each cup of coffee, tea, soda, or fruit juice you drink daily. Then, add another 8 ounces for each half hour you exercise. As the numbers add up, it makes sense that dehydration is so common.

According to these rules, most people are dehydrated, and you're an exceptional person if you already drink the proper amount of water daily. But who can drink all that water daily without guzzling? I have a tip that will maximize your effort.

- The best way to prevent dehydration is to sip your water. When you sip your water it's more likely to absorb into your tissues. When you drink you're water down quickly it's more likely to go straight to the kidneys and cause frequent urination.

The Water Wars

There is so much conflicting information regarding what type of water you should drink. Some say filtered water, some say alkaline water, some say spring water, and some say distilled water, or even reverse osmosis. There is one thing that I know for certain: I don't hear anyone these days touting the benefits of tap water.

Personally I prefer to drink water that's filtered with minerals. Our ancestors have been drinking water from springs and rivers since the beginning of our history, but those rivers and springs were not polluted like they are today.

If you have access to filtered water or alkaline water, definitely choose that. Drink filtered water that is free of chlorine, microorganisms, solvents, and heavy metals. Mineral water (as compared to distilled water) is believed to prevent the leaching of minerals from the body.

But the true goals today are to prevent dehydration and to get you to drink more water. Since many people don't care for the taste of water, primarily caused by the over-saturation of sugary drinks, I want to emphasize the goal is to drink water in its pure form, not to drink liquid.

Here are two recommendations to help get the palate used to tasting water:

1. If you don't like the taste of water, squeeze a little fresh lemon juice into your water daily until your body develops a taste for water.

2. Don't drink any other beverages for the entire day until you've consumed your complete daily water intake.

Practicing those two simple steps will immediately improve your water intake and your health. You will feel better, be more energized, and save a little money, too.

Chapter 5

Solution # 2:
Nature's Stress Relief: The Healing Power of Vitamins, Minerals, Herbs, Essential Oils, and Water

"Take care of your body. It's the only place you have to live."
~ Jim Rohn

Everyone needs adequate micronutrients (vitamins, minerals, enzymes, and trace elements) for good health. Ideally, you would be able to obtain all the necessary micronutrients from a well-balanced diet. However, the nutritional quality of the food in this society has been steadily declining, particularly in the last century.

In the past, people ate foods that were whole, fresh, in season, and locally grown in nutrient-dense soil. Now, most foods are refined, preserved, and grown in nutrient-depleted soils, making it difficult for you to get all the nutrients you need solely from food, no matter how "nutritious" your diet may seem.

Since stress, activity level, medications, and illnesses can increase your need for vitamins and minerals, nutritional supplements may be needed to bridge the gap between your diet and your actual vitamin/mineral requirements. But supplements aren't a cure-all. They're designed to supplement—*to "add to" your diet*—not to replace your food. They're great as an addition to your diet and if prescribed they should be taken regularly.

Nutrients have been shown to have many beneficial, preventative, and therapeutic effects on disease, and in particular stress-related conditions. The body benefits from the use of vitamins, minerals, herbs, essential oils, and water treatments in many ways. This chapter will help you understand these treatments to reduce your stress.

Vitamins and Minerals

There are many foods that can be eaten regularly that are helpful in meeting the demands of stress. In the previous chapter you learned many food solutions to maintain health, but certain nutrients specifically have been found to be beneficial in relieving stress.

Vitamins A and B-complex, calcium, potassium, and magnesium help reduce the feelings of irritability and anxiety. People with high levels of Vitamin C do not show the expected mental and physical signs of stress when they undergo acute stressful situations, and they bounce back from stressful situations faster. Vitamin C is especially good for your adrenal glands.

Vitamin E protects cellular stress, or what is called oxidative stress or free radical cell damage. Selenium is a powerful antioxidant that works with Vitamin E to reduce cell damage and oxidative stress.

Zinc works with your metabolism, and iron is a part of your red blood cells and helps transport oxygen to exercising muscles. If either zinc or iron is low, this will contribute to fatigue.

An element of Vitamin B-complex, pantothenic acid (B5) is especially important in preventing stress. It has a deep effect on the adrenal glands and the immune system. Adequate amounts of B5 can help prevent many changes caused by stress.

Calcium is a natural sedative. Deficiencies can cause fatigue, nervousness, and tension. Magnesium is known as nature's tranquilliser, it's a great muscle relaxer, and it has been associated with the prevention of heart attacks. Magnesium deficiencies may lead to excitability, irritability, apprehension, and emotional disorders. Magnesium is also necessary for the absorption of calcium and potassium.

Chapter 5: Solution # 2: Nature's Stress Relief: The Healing Power of Vitamins, Mineral, Herbs, Essential Oils, and Water

Potassium deficiencies are associated with breathlessness, fatigue, insomnia, and low blood sugar. Potassium is essential for healthy heart muscles.

Here is a list of the food sources of vitamins and minerals needed to reduce stress:

- **Vitamin A:** green, orange, and yellow vegetables, liver, cod-liver oil, eggs, dairy products

- **Vitamin B-complex:** cashews, green leafy vegetables, yeast, sprouts, bananas
    - **B1 (thiamine):** wheat germ, whole wheat, peas, beans, enriched flour, fish, peanuts, meat
    - **B2 (riboflavin):** Dairy products, eggs, and meat are the main sources of vitamin B2. Leafy green vegetables, whole grains, and enriched grains contain some Vitamin B2.
    - **B3 (niacin/niacinamide):** peanuts, brewer's yeast, fish, meat; whole grains contain some Vitamin B3
    - **B5 (pantothenic acid):** Liver, yeast, and salmon are the best sources of pantothenic acid. It is also found in most other foods, including vegetables, dairy, eggs, grains, and meat.
    - **B6 (pyridoxine):** wheat bran, beans/lentils, sunflower seeds, walnuts, cashews, avocado, potatoes, bananas, tuna
    - **Folic acid:** yeast, liver, uncooked vegetables, leafy green vegetables, beans, peas, citrus fruits, beets, lentils, avocado, nuts, seeds., asparagus, broccoli, wheat germ, meat
    - **B12:** all foods of animal origin, including dairy, eggs, meat, poultry, and fish. Small, inconsistent amounts occur in seaweed (including nori and chlorella) and tempeh.

- **Vitamin C:** black currants, broccoli, Brussels sprouts, cauliflower, strawberries, citrus fruit, spinach, red peppers, parsley, potatoes, and tomatoes.

- **Vitamin E:** wheat germ oil, nuts and seeds, whole grains, egg yolks, and leafy green vegetables. Certain vegetable oils (corn oil, soybean oil, safflower oil, sunflower oil) should contain significant amounts of Vitamin E.
- **Calcium:** seeds such as alfalfa, sunflower seeds, pumpkin, sprouts, almonds, dairy products, sardines, canned salmon, broccoli, green leafy vegetables
- **Essential fatty acids:** fish that live in cold, deep water (salmon, halibut, mackerel, herring, sardines, etc.), canola oil, flaxseed oil, walnut oil, raw nuts, seeds and legumes, borage oil, grape seed oil, primrose oil, sesame oil, soybean oil
- **Magnesium:** nuts, grains, beans, dark green vegetables, fish, meats, fruits, vegetables, seeds, dates, prunes
- **Iron:** oysters, meat, poultry, fish, dried fruit, molasses, leafy green vegetables, wine, acidic foods (such as tomato sauce) cooked in an iron pan
- **Potassium:** bananas, nuts, unrefined grains
- **Selenium:** Brazil nuts, yeast, whole grains, seafood
- **Zinc:** oysters, meat, eggs, seafood, black-eyed peas, tofu, wheat germ, whole grains

Herbal Medicine

Herbal medicine has been used for ages as a means of treating and preventing disease. Herbal medicine can be used to treat, manage, and minimize the effects of stress. Compared to conventional medicines (primarily drugs), herbal medicines are less expensive, are readily available, have minimal side effects, and tend to offer long-lasting benefits in terms of overall wellness.

The best class of herbs for supporting and reinvigorating your adrenals are adaptogenic. An adaptogen is any substance that helps the body function more towards its normal level. For example, if

Chapter 5: Solution # 2: Nature's Stress Relief: The Healing Power of Vitamins, Mineral, Herbs, Essential Oils, and Water

cortisol is too high, an adaptogen will lower it; and if it's too low, it will raise it. Adaptogens have a normalizing effect on the adrenal glands. They revitalize fatigued adrenals without over-stimulating them and help the body cope more effectively with stress.

Nervines are a class of herbs that have a beneficial affect on the nervous system. The effect on the nervous system can be toning or strengthening, calming, or stimulating to the nervous system. Since stress is not easily defined by its effect on your body, herbs that can shift their action based on your instantaneous needs are best for treatment. That's why adaptogens and nervines are commonly used.

Common Herb to Treat Stress

- Ashwagandha (*Withania somnifera*): traditionally prescribed as a tonic for all kinds of weaknesses, as well as to promote strength and vigor; adaptogenic, anti-inflammatory.

- Siberian ginseng root (*Eleutherococcus senticosus*): increases your stamina, helps to reduce external stress, increases immunity to stress and recovery time, supports and rejuvenates adrenal function, increase resistance to stress, normalizes metabolism, counteracts mental fatigue, and is known to increase and sustain energy levels, physical stamina, and endurance. It has antidepressant properties, calms anxiousness, improves sleep, diminishes lethargy, lessens irritability, and induces a feeling of well-being.

- Licorice root (*Glycyrrhiza glabra*): best known for supporting adrenal function. This anti-stress herb is known to increase energy, endurance, and vitality; used to ease drug withdrawal; is used as an anti-inflammatory; and fortifies cortisol levels. It may increases blood pressure, so those of you with high blood pressure should use caution when taking licorice in high doses for extended periods of time.

- Golden Root (*Rhodiola rosea*): enhances your ability

to tolerate stress, and helps to calm an overactive stress response system and replenish depleted energy reserves.

- Maca (*Lepidium peruvianum*): ability to increase stamina, energy, and endurance, and improves the ability to withstand stress. This adaptogenic herb helps normalize the body's response to stress, modulate cortisol levels, reduce the exhaustion that follows a stressful event, and protect the body against the negative effects of stress.

- Hops (*Humulus lupulus*): relaxing and strengthening to the nerves; relaxes tension, relieves anxiety, is fast-acting, produces sleep, is used to decrease the desire for alcohol.

- Lobelia (*Lobelia laxiflora*): has a beneficial effect on the whole body, is powerful relaxant in many diseases, balances the glands, is valuable in stress crisis, is effective in causing immediate relaxation, and is powerful in removing disease and promoting health.

- Scullcap (*Scutellaria lateriflora*): one of the best nerve tonics; very quieting and soothing to the nerves of worry and restlessness; good in neuralgia, aches, and pains; useful with drug and alcohol withdrawal; has detoxification properties.

- Valerian (*Valeriana officinalis*): nourishing and soothing to the nervous system, useful in hysterics, can serve as a substitute for valium to overcome addiction, helps reduce anxiety, tension, insomnia, and muscle spasms.

- Lady's slipper (*Cypripedium pubescens*): rebuilds damaged and frayed nerves; excellent for nervous headaches and irritability; helpful for all stress, tension, and anxiety states; enhances calming and easing of the mind.

- Passion flower (*Passiflora incarnata*): sedative, antispasmodic, tranquilizing, helps insomnia, reduces nervous over-activity and panic.

Chapter 5: Solution # 2: Nature's Stress Relief: The Healing Power of Vitamins, Mineral, Herbs, Essential Oils, and Water

- Black cohosh (*Cimicifuga racemosa*): helpful with nervous disorders, excellent remedy for high blood pressure, helpful in epileptic seizures, dizziness, convulsions, contains antibacterial properties to calm nerves and relieve muscular pain.

- St. John's wort (*Hypericum perforatum*): nervine, sedative, powerful blood purifier, good in hysteria and nervous affections, useful for chronic fatigue syndrome and mental burnout, anti-inflammatory.

- Chamomile (*Matricaria recutita*): contains tryptophan, which works in the body to induce natural sleep, helpful to the nerves.

- Blue vervain (*Verbena hastata*): relaxes the nerves; useful in sleeplessness, nervousness, and nervous headache; a natural tranquilizer; produces an overall feeling of well-being.

- Oats (*Avena sativa*): full of Vitamin B; work as nervine relaxants to ease tension and strengthen and support the nervous system, and as a tonic to promote energy to handle the stress and depression; can also be helpful in relieving exhaustion.

- Lemon balm (*Melissa officinalis*): promotes relaxation and relieves stress; possesses sedative/tranquilizing effects, anti-gas, fever-reducing, antibacterial, memory-enhancing.

Herbs for Stress Relief

While many of these herbs may sound familiar, it may be confusing to know where to find them and how to take them. I would caution you to know that, although herbs are natural, they are still very powerful. Always seek the advice of a professional before taking them.

Many herbs are sold in health food stores as individual herbs or premixed formulas. You may see a "calm formula" and/or "adrenal support formula" on the store shelves. If you need general support, these formulas can be helpful. Also, more herbs can be purchased from online sources. In either case, please always opt for the highest quality possible.

You can also buy herbs in liquid form (tinctures) or tea form. This would be the dried leaf, root, or aerial parts. When herbs are purchased individually, it allows for more flexibility in making and changing your formula to meet your specific needs.

Simply making and smelling herbal teas can have a calming effect on you, and some people drink teas just for the ritual of it. If you get confused, discuss your choice of herbs with a health food store employee, or, better yet, have a trained naturopathic physician or herbalist create a formula perfect for you.

Aromatherapy

Stress causes an interesting array of emotions. You can fluctuate from anger to sadness, from anxiety to irritability, and from nervousness to fear. As a stress reliever, aromatherapy can be used quite successfully. Aromatherapy as a natural, healing modality is under-utilized in today's society, especially since it's so powerful and relatively inexpensive.

Aromatherapy uses the sense of smell. Humans have the capability to distinguish 10,000 different smells, which can have a profound effect on the human mind and body. Essential oils are extracted from aromatic plants and made of chemical compositions that, when they reach your brain, can exert specific effects on your mind and body.

Smell stimulates the part of your brain that controls your emotions, moods, memory, and learning (the cerebrum). Smell reaches the olfactory (smelling) nerves in the brain via cilia, which are the fine hair lining the nose. This is the basis of the aromatherapy.

In addition, by rubbing and massaging the oil on the skin, essential oils can be applied directly to the muscles, ligaments, etc.

Chapter 5: Solution # 2: Nature's Stress Relief: The Healing Power of Vitamins, Mineral, Herbs, Essential Oils, and Water

Other than rubbing and massaging, they can be inhaled, sprayed on objects or in the air, and dropped in water used for soaking. Each essential oil has its own healing property. Here are examples of essential oils that are used for relieving stress:

- Basil: useful in cases of mental and intellectual fatigue, negativity, or burnout; helps improve your concentration, clarity, and enthusiasm

- Bergamot: encouraging; good for anxiety, depression, emotional imbalance, despondency, concentration, motivation

- Cedarwood: aids focus, concentration, strength of purpose, and stability; is particularly useful against mental strain, worry, and anxiety

- Cinnamon: invigorating and aids positivity; helps fight stress and fatigue

- Clary sage: calming and uplifting; promotes feelings of well-being; calms the nerves and reduces stress; promotes concentration when used in inhalation therapy

- Eucalyptus: used to combat confusion, sluggishness, and restlessness; aids confidence, balance, enthusiasm, vitality, creativity, regeneration, and understanding

- Frankincense: good for exhaustion, panic attacks, anxiety, nervous tension, and other stress-related disorders; calms the mind; provides inspiration and emotional stability

- Geranium: good for acute fear, extreme mood swings, balance, tranquility, humor, nervous tension, and other stress-related disorders

- German chamomile: good for irritation, impatience, nervous tension, and other stress-related disorders

- Grapefruit: a mental stimulator; can be used to counteract mental pressure/exhaustion and frustration, and improve clarity, balance, positivity, and inspiration

Stop Stressing Me Out

- Jasmine: emotionally warming; uplifts, nurtures, and boosts confidence; good for depression and other stress-related disorders, and addiction
- Lavender: particularly useful in stressful situations; has been shown to reduce levels of anxiety, depression, and fatigue; aids clarity, balance, relaxation, and rejuvenation
- Lemongrass: helps reduce stress and panic; improves concentration and focus
- Marjoram: effective relieving stress and helping insomnia
- Melissa (lemon balm): promotes relaxation and relieves stress; possesses sedative/tranquilizing qualities; powerful antiviral
- Orange: provides mental stimulation; helps fight apathy, anxiety and burnout
- Peppermint: clarifying; good for mental fatigue, overwork, apathy, concentration, and vitality
- Pine: good for combating stress and a lack of confidence, and providing assurance and balance
- Roman chamomile: good for irritation, impatience, nervous tension, and other stress-related disorders
- Rose: soothing, uplifting; creates a sense of well-being; good for depression, nervous tension, and other stress-related disorders
- Rosemary: aids energy, creativity, clarity, and concentration; is useful in cases of strain, overwork, fatigue, sluggishness, lethargy
- Sandalwood: comforting; soothes anxiety, tension, or stress; restores the spirit; relaxing; good for depression and other stress-related disorders

Chapter 5: Solution # 2: Nature's Stress Relief: The Healing Power of Vitamins, Mineral, Herbs, Essential Oils, and Water

- Ylang ylang: uplifting, calming, balancing; good for anxiety, nervous tension, depression, stress-related disorders, impatience, and fear

Dr. Lisa Lewis's Stop Stressing Me Out Formula

Ingredients:
5 drops bergamot essential oil
5 drops frankincense essential oil
3 drops lavender
3 drops orange
3 drops marjoram
1 drop jasmine *or* ylang ylang essential oil
1 drop chamomile
1/4 cup (60ml) carrier oil of your choice (olive, almond, jojoba, or grapeseed oil)

Method:
Combine all ingredients in a dark glass dropper bottle.
Let stand for 24 hours to blend completely before using.
Store the bottle in a cool, dark place.

To use, take three long, slow, deep breaths of the aroma. Take a short break, then take three more deep breaths. Repeat the cycle three times.
You can massage the oil directly into your temples, or place a drop on a cotton ball or on your pillow case as desired.
It can also be used as a lotion or bath oil.

Water Therapy: Hydrotherapy

Water has been used for thousands of years as a method of healing the body. Hydrotherapy is defined as using water to eliminate waste from the body, and to maintain, relieve, and restore health. The beauty of hydrotherapy is that many treatments

Stop Stressing Me Out

can be done in your home, although spas and other facilities also specialize in hydrotherapy treatments.

Water is an amazing substance for healing for several reasons:

1. Water can store and carry heat and energy.
2. Water is used in many forms, from ice to steam.
3. Water can dissolve other substances.
4. Water cannot hurt you even if you are allergic to many things, and water can help blood flow.
5. Hot water is considered relaxing, and opens the blood vessels to increase flow and remove waste from the body.
6. Cold water is stimulating, causing blood vessels to constrict and direct blood flow to the internal organs.

Types of Hydrotherapy

There are several different types of hydrotherapy, some of which are:

- Hot and cold compresses: help relieve pain and boost the immune system
  - o Fomentation: Treats acute conditions such as chest colds and can also shorten the length of the illness. Place a hot compress on the chest and a cold compress on the forehead.
- Steam bath: uses moisture (steam) and heat to cleanse the body and soothe muscle
- Dry heat sauna: uses dry heat to promote sweating, detoxification, and muscle relaxation
- Sitz bath: Soak in a bath of warm water for 30 minutes or so. You can add Epsom salt, mineral mud, dead sea salts, ginger, essentials oils, etc. Sitz baths can be used for pain, PMS, cystitis, polyps, etc.
- Wet sock treatment: Before bed place white, cold, wet socks

Chapter 5: Solution # 2: Nature's Stress Relief: The Healing Power of Vitamins, Mineral, Herbs, Essential Oils, and Water

on your feet, then cover with another pair of dry socks. Leave on overnight. The process of warming and drying the sock stimulates your immune system. It's a good way to get rid of fevers, sore throats, ear infections, headaches, nasal congestion, coughs, and sinus infections.

Two Important Types of Hydrotherapy

Contrast Hydrotherapy

In many cases, cold and hot treatments are used together in the course of a treatment. Alternating applications of hot and cold water are used to change blood flow and release muscle tension. Contrast hydrotherapy has been used to help relieve headaches, boost your immune system, and treat musculoskeletal problems.

Colonic Hydrotherapy (Colonics)

Colonic hydrotherapy uses water to gently cleanse the large intestine or colon. In the past, colonics have been called "high enemas" because of their ability to cleanse the colon entirely, including the ascending colon and cecum.

Colonics are used to cleanse the body of toxins that build up in the colon. When these toxins can no longer be effectively eliminated from the large intestine, they can cause autointoxication (the poisoning of one's own system through toxin buildup).

Toxin buildup results in a wide variety of symptoms, which may include aching joints, headaches, poor concentration, mood swings, PMS, lethargy, and fatigue. Many diseases may also be linked to autointoxication.

Colonics themselves are not a cure for any disease, but they can aid the body's natural ability to heal itself by temporarily removing the overload on the system caused by the toxins.

Using these natural tools should help treat both the symptoms and results of stress. They can also strengthen your resolve to begin handling the true underlining causes of your stress. In either case, your stress can reduce significantly and quickly, so start today.

Chapter 6

Solution #3:
Acupuncture—The Stress Reliever : No Pain...All Gain

"Acupuncture offers the possibility of a deep healing transformation on a mind, body and spirit level!"

"Acupuncture can bring us a deep sense of peace and well-being."

Stress Relief

A common response from patients when asked the question "What would you like to achieve with this acupuncture treatment?" is "I have too much stress. I need to reduce my stress!"

When asking about behaviors used to get through the day or night, these are common statements I hear from my patients:

"I need a glass of wine or two at night to unwind before bed."

"I grab a cigarette when I'm trying to relax, sometimes with a drink. I like to light up when I'm drinking."

"I need my coffee in the morning. Without it I would never make it to work."

"I drink coffee every day, but I'm not addicted. I really love how it tastes and or smells."

"I keep candy in my drawer at work, my glove compartment, and my pocketbook. I get really tired around 3:00 p.m. and on the drive home from work, sugar lifts me up."

Stop Stressing Me Out

"I'm tired all day—exhausted even, but I can't fall asleep when I lay down at night."

"I'm an emotional eater. When I'm upset or sad, I just eat. I can't help myself."

There's no standard formula to help relieve stress. Commonly, people resort to quick fixes (alcohol, cigarettes, sugar, and all sorts of over-the-counter and prescription drugs) to cope with stress, tension, and strain in your life. Many times these coping mechanisms are conscious, but mostly they are subconscious.

Food can also be used to cope with stress and emotional discomfort. People may eat when they feel anxious, depressed, and stressed.

There is no magic stress-reduction pill, nor do alcohol, sleeping tablets, and antidepressants offer any real solution to reducing stress. Antidepressants, although often prescribed to reduce stress, offer limited short-term relief at best and, at worst, can cause dependence.

What Is Acupuncture, and Can it Help Me?

Stress. Everyone has it. The question is: How do you get rid of it? One strategy that works wonders is acupuncture. It's amazing for stress relief, but many people don't understand acupuncture and how it works. This chapter will provide insight into this ancient practice.

Acupuncture is based on the concept that the physical, spiritual, and emotional bodies are connected in function. A network of energy called Qi (pronounced "chee") flows through all aspects of the body. The goal of acupuncture is to regulate and balance your life force—the body energy or Qi.

Qi flows through the body in channels called meridians. Acupuncture uses very thin stainless-steel needles to stimulate specific points along the meridians. This stimulation can unblock energy that is "stuck," or to bring energy into areas that are lacking energy, allowing the body to move back into balance.

Acupuncture has a number of beneficial effects, which creates

Chapter 6: Solution # 3: Acupuncture—The Stress Reliever: No Pain...All Gain

a relaxation response. This relaxation response can decrease your heart rate, lower your blood pressure, reduce your stress, increase your energy, and improve your tissue regeneration capacity, helping you heal faster.

Most of my patients have felt the calming or tranquilizing action that is of particular interest for stress reduction. Acupuncture can also relieve feelings of anxiety and depression, which may be serious handicaps when coping with difficult life situations, domestic, and social and work problems.

Symptoms of stress can be an imbalance of vital body energy that can be corrected by acupuncture treatment. My patients usually begin to feel more energetic after their first acupuncture treatment and much improved with six or so treatments, unless they are suffering from a debilitating disease.

Acupuncture can give you a feeling of well-being and self-confidence. It is an effective substitute for sleeping pills, tranquilizers, and antidepressant drugs. Acupuncture can be used in many cases, not only as an alternative to these drugs but also to treat side effects and dependence. In fact, a number of my patients have come for acupuncture treatment specifically to taper off their antidepressants.

There is considerable evidence that after acupuncture treatments, people have substantially reduce the consumption of drugs, especially antidepressants. Does this sound like you? If so, acupuncture may help you, too.

Acupuncture can provide a safe and effective tool to reduce your stress. It will not, of course, change your life circumstances, but it will usually produce a feeling of well-being. I have also experienced patients who became stronger, both mentally and physically after receiving successive acupuncture treatments.. Because of their renewed strength and clarity of mind, they were able to lift themselves out of situations that seemed impossible before treatment.

Acupuncture can open your window of opportunity. As your heavy feelings of stress are relieved, you feel more confidence in your ability to cope with unpleasant aspects of your life situation and strong enough to make the necessary changes.

Is Acupuncture Safe?

Acupuncture is considered very safe. While it's a medical procedure that punctures the skin and underlying tissues, injuries and side effects are very rare, and if they do occur, they're usually minor. Sterile acupuncture needles are required by law. Most acupuncture clinics use sterile, one-use, disposable needles.

Does it Hurt?

Acupuncture is considered to be relatively painless. However, with correct stimulation, you may feel the movement of Qi. The Qi sensations vary widely and may be described as heaviness, distention, tingling, or electric. You may feel these sensations only at the location of the needle, or traveling up or down the meridian. These sensations are a sign that your Qi is adjusting toward balance.

Patients commonly fall asleep after the needles have been inserted. They sleep very soundly; many even snore loudly. When the treatment is over, I wake them and they always ask, "How long was I asleep?" I usually answer that they were asleep about 20–35 minutes.

They say,

"Wow, that was the best sleep I've had in months, maybe years. It feels like I was asleep for hours.

I feel so relaxed, I don't want to get up.

It feels like I had a two hour massage."

That's how the body and mind feel when they're in balance. Isn't that amazing?

Stress Is Liver Qi Stagnation

In this medicine the main function of the liver is to ensure smooth flow of Qi. This is the most important of all the liver functions, and it is central to nearly all liver problems. This is one of the most common problems that I see in practice.

Chapter 6: Solution # 3: Acupuncture—The Stress Reliever: No Pain...All Gain

What does it mean that the liver ensures smooth flow of Qi? This literally means "to flow" and "to let out." Many books explain this function by using terms like *disperse, extend, loosen, relax, make smooth and free,* and *circulate.* So, the liver ensures that there is a smooth flow of energy, Qi, throughout the entire body, in all organs and in all directions.

There are three aspects to this function:

1. The liver function has a deep influence on the emotional state. If your function is normal, Qi flows normally and your emotional life is happy. If not, your circulation obstructed and your Qi becomes restrained.

   Your emotional symptoms would be frustration, depression, or repressed anger. Your physical symptoms would be hypochondriac (left or right side of the upper abdomen) pain, sensation of oppression in your chest, a feeling of "lump" in your throat, or abdominal distension.

   In women, it may cause premenstrual tension, including depression, irritability, and breast distension and tenderness.

2. The smooth flow of liver Qi assists digestive function. If liver Qi flows smoothly, your food can digest easily and efficiently. If not and your liver Qi becomes stuck, you may experience belching, sour regurgitation, nausea, vomiting, or diarrhea.

3. The smooth flow of Qi affects your bile flow. If liver Qi is stuck, your bile flow may be obstructed, causing a bitter taste in your mouth, belching, or jaundice.

In relation to liver Qi, the most important and common pattern is that of stagnation of liver Qi. The most striking and apparent symptom of liver Qi stagnation is distension. This shows up as a feeling of distension, bloating, or fullness of the upper, middle, and lower abdomen.

Anger is the emotion that is most related to liver function. *Anger* is a broad term used that includes feelings of frustration, repressed anger, resentment, and irritation.

If your liver is functioning well and its Qi is flowing smoothly, your emotional state is happy and easy-going. You are in good spirits and freely expressing your emotions. If not, you will express anger and irritability. Over a long period of time, you could experience constant resentment, repressed anger, or depression.

On a physical level, your constrained emotions could be "carried" in your chest, hypochondrium, epigastrium (upper center of the abdomen), or throat. You will experience a feeling of tightness of the chest and perhaps sigh frequently, distension/fullness of the hypogastrium (lower abdomen), tension in the stomach, or a feeling of a lump in your throat with difficulty swallowing.

Treatment of Liver Qi Stagnation

Symptoms

- Feeling of distension of hypochondrium and chest, hypochondriac pain, sighing, hiccup.

- Melancholy, depression, moodiness, changes in your mental state.

- Nausea, vomiting, epigastric pain, poor appetite, sour regurgitation, belching, feeling of pulsation in epigastrium, churning feeling in the stomach, abdominal distension, borborygmi (increased stomach sounds), diarrhea.

- Unhappiness, feeling "wound up," feeling of lump in your throat, feeling of difficulty in swallowing.

- Irregular periods, painful periods, distension of breasts before the periods, premenstrual tension, and irritability.

Treatment
Principle of treatment: disperse the Liver and regulate Qi.
Acupuncture Points: GB-34, LIV-3, LIV-13, LIV-14, SJ-6, P-6.

Chapter 6: Solution # 3: Acupuncture—The Stress Reliever: No Pain...All Gain

Diet

If you eat an excessive amount of greasy and "hot" foods, this can cause liver Qi stagnation. Chinese dietary principles define hot foods as lamb, beef, curries, spices, and alcohol. Deep-fried foods are also considered hot. These foods should be eaten minimally or avoided.

Chinese Herbal Formulas

There are several Chinese herbal formulas developed to treat liver Qi stagnation, but each formula is very specific to the symptoms you are experiencing. The four formulas listed here are the most common. Each lists the signs and symptoms you need to experience for the herbal formula to be indicated for you.

Xiao Yao San
Si Ni San
Chai Hu Shu Gan Tang
Yue Ju Wan

Xiao Yao Tang (Most Common)

Clinical Signs and Symptoms: Stress, hypochondriac pain, depression, irritability, insomnia, bitter taste in mouth, fatigue, dry mouth and throat, headache, dizziness, anemia, poor appetite. Breast distention, cysts or pain, alternating fever and chills, alternating diarrhea and constipation, irregular menstruation, dysmenorrhea, PMS. Gastritis, and stress-induced ulcers.

Case Study #1

A 36-year-old woman suffers from irregular periods, which have a very light flow, and she has dysmenorrhea (painful periods) for the first day or so of her cycle. She noticed that her skin and hair are drier than normal and says she's been wearing more makeup since her complexion looks more dull than usual.

She feels distension in both her abdomen and breasts, which are worse a few days before her period. She suffers from moodiness and mild depression, which are also worse just before her period. She also complains that her hands feel cold all the time.

She has a really stressful job, which also causes her to travel two to three days per week. As a result she is tired and has difficulty sleeping, but it could be a result of changing time zones frequently. She notices a feeling of a lump in her throat when her stress level is really high.

After checking her pulse and tongue (part of the diagnostic process), she was given the herbal formula Xiao Yao Tang. This is one of the most common herbal formulas for stress, especially for women. Its primary purpose is to soothe liver Qi and release the depressed Qi.

Si Ni San

Clinical Signs and Symptoms: Cold fingers and toes although the body is warm, sometimes accompanied by the sensation of irritability and fullness in the chest and epigastrium. There may be abdominal pain and/or severe diarrhea.

Si Ni San is great for stress, similar to Xiao Yao San except it's more specific for stress with digestive challenges and cold fingers and/ or toes.

Chai Hu Shu Gan Tang

Clinical Signs and Symptoms: Depression, hypochondriac distension or pain, a fullness sensation in the chest, belching, painful menstruation, breast distension, or alternating chills and fever.

Case Study #2

A 44-year-old man has symptoms of uncontrolled belching. He says his wife complains about it and kids think it's funny, but it really causes him embarrassment. The belching was preceded by nausea and hiccups for about three months.

His wife and coworkers complain that he's very irritable and snappy, and he feels like he's been withdrawing slightly from

Chapter 6: Solution # 3: Acupuncture—The Stress Reliever: No Pain...All Gain

interaction. He has been working long hours and eating fast food almost every meal, which he says makes the belching worse.

After pulse and tongue diagnosis, this patient was given Chai Hu Shu Gan Tang. The most common symptoms for choosing Chai Hu Shu Gan Tang are belching and irritability, along with proper pulse and tongue diagnosis.

Yue Ju Wan

Clinical Signs and Symptoms: Focal distension, a stifling sensation in the chest and abdomen, fixed pain in the hypochondria, belching, vomiting, acid regurgitation, mild coughing with copious sputum, reduced appetite, and indigestion.

Case Study #3

A 32-year-old female presents with chronic gall bladder pain that she's had for two years. She has pain in her right hypochondrium, sour belching, nausea, distension, and an oppressive feeling in her chest and abdomen, which gets worse with greasy foods. She occasionally vomits up her food which temporarily relieves the pain.

Her primary care doctor keeps suggesting surgery, but she doesn't want to go under the knife—mostly for vanity reasons because she likes wearing a bikini and doesn't want a scar on her abdomen.

She has a very intense personality and has a high-stress job in the legal field. She knows she can't keep putting off the surgery because the pain is getting worse, but she wants more options. Meanwhile, her pain and her stress keep increasing.

Along with a pulse and tongue diagnosis, she was given Yue Ju Wan. This formula is designed to improve Qi circulation and relieve stagnation. The key indicating symptoms are fixed pain, indigestion, and vomiting.

Chapter 7

Solution #4:
Breath of Life—Deep Breathing, Meditation, and Relaxation Strategies

"When you own your breath, nobody can steal your peace."
~ Author Unknown

Relaxation techniques can be considered the most common and well-known approaches to stress reduction. The beauty of these techniques is that they are easy to learn and easy to do. But just like anything else in life, these techniques only work when they're actually used.

Another wonderful aspect of these techniques is that they take relatively little time—and create big results. So you can get a big bang for your buck. With just a few minutes a day, or an hour, you can reap high rewards.

I know you hear this all the time: "Rock-hard abs in just 10 minutes a day," "the five-minute workout," "lose a dress size in three days," etc. Someone is always trying to convince you that you can have everything you dreamed of in a few minutes a day.

So, why should you believe that relaxation techniques work to reduce stress in just a few minutes or an hour a day? They are designed to control and relax the body and release stress, as well as control the organ systems in the body. Practicing them daily provides a cumulative affect of relaxation and stress relief.

A few of these relaxation techniques include:

- Deep / belly breathing or breath work

- Meditation
- Progressive muscle relaxation
- Visualization
- Journaling

Most are easy to learn. You will need to practice these techniques often, so you can learn them thoroughly. Since they are new approaches to stress reduction, they will eventually become conditioned responses. You'll find yourself doing the techniques without even thinking about it. They will provide natural, daily, even continuous stress relief.

You can choose to adopt the habit rule. Some say it takes 21 days, and others say it take 66 days to develop a habit. It all depends on the difficulty of the challenge, but I suggest you be like Nike and "just do it."

Don't put undue stress on yourself with a timetable and rules. If the techniques resonate with you, you will begin to crave them, like food. Find a few moments each day and you'll feel the benefit.

Deep/Belly Breathing

> "Sometimes the most important thing in a whole day is the rest we take between two deep breaths."
> *~ Etty Hillesum*

How you breathe has a profound effect on your life and health. Not only does it change how much oxygen is going into your body and how much waste is coming out of your body, but it also affects heart function, immune system function, mood, stress levels, hormone levels, digestion, strength, endurance, and a wide variety of other things. In short, how you breathe can influence almost every aspect of your health and well-being.

The most efficient way to breathe is diaphragmatic breathing, or belly breathing. This is the most common form of breathing in

Chapter 7: Solution # 4: Breath of Life—Deep Breathing, Meditation, and Relaxation Strategies

healthy infants and young children, but as people get older they tend to breathe using their chest and shoulder muscles and less of their diaphragm.

Take a deep breath in and out. Did you feel your chest expand and contract? Did your shoulders go up as you drew air into your lungs? This is the way many adults breathe. To breathe more efficiently, and in a way that promotes relaxation, let's look at how you probably breathe while you're asleep.

Typically, when in a relaxed sleeping state, you breathe from your diaphragm, the muscle between the abdomen and the chest. The chest does not obviously move in and out, and the shoulders do not move up and down.

Instead, the abdomen rises with each breath you inhale and lowers with each breath you exhale. It is both more effortless and more efficient than the typical waking approach to breathing—and, as a result, it's more relaxing.

How can you practice relaxed/belly breathing?

Exercise

Lie on your back on a bed or recliner. Place your feet slightly apart and lightly rest one hand on your abdomen, just near your navel. Rest your other hand on your chest.

Inhale through your nose and exhale through your mouth. Breathe in, using the diaphragm, pushing the abdomen out, completely filling you lower and upper lungs.

Calmly exhale most of the air in your lungs. With each breath you take, focus on your breathing and recognize which hand is moving.

Repeat this exercise for five to 15 minutes each day.

If you practice relaxed/belly breathing regularly it can again become second nature to you, naturally reduce your tension, and improve your circulation.

Alternating Nostril Breathing

The alternating nostril breathing technique is especially good

Stop Stressing Me Out

for those who suffer from chronic sinusitis, allergies, and lung infections.

Exercise

Press the thumb of your left hand against the left side of your nose blocking the air passage. Breathe in through your right nostril for a count of 10.

Move your hand so that the side of your index finger closes the air passage on the right side of your nose. Breathe out of the left nostril for a count of 10.

Switch hands. Breathe in through the left nostril and out through the right nostril for a count of 10.

Breathing Colors

Breathing colors is a combination of meditation and breathing. It is especially helpful for relaxation, stress reduction, high blood pressure, generalized immune stimulation, and insomnia.

Bend your knees and straighten your legs. Each time you straighten your legs to come up, breathe in. As you breathe in, you will breathe in colors from the earth/rainbow (red, orange, yellow, green, blue, indigo, violet, and white) and the air through your feet and hands. Each time you bend your knees to go down, breathe out. As you breathe out, let the colors go back into your environment.

Remember: Both the alternate nostril breathing and breathing colors techniques are great for relaxation and powerful stress relievers. Breathing colors is great for reducing high blood pressure, boosting your immune system, and insomnia, while the alternating nostril techniques is great for chronic sinus infections, allergies, and lung infections.

The "Relaxation Response" Technique

"The mark of a successful man is one that has spent an entire day on the bank of a river without feeling guilty about it."
~ Author Unknown

Chapter 7: Solution # 4: Breath of Life—Deep Breathing, Meditation, and Relaxation Strategies

Recognizing that some people who practice meditation are capable of reducing their heart rate, blood pressure, and oxygen consumption, Relaxation Response is a simple practice that focuses on the qualities in meditation that create a sense of relaxation and stress reduction.

Here's how to do it:

Exercise

Every day, plan to spend some time at rest (not asleep). Close your eyes and relax your muscles. Then focus on your breathing, making it deep/belly breathing and very regular.

Then continuously repeat one word. You can repeat the word aloud or in your mind. It should be either a simple word such as *relax* or *easy,* a religious word or phrase, a brief phrase that has no meaning (such as the *ohm* used in transcendental meditation), or one that simply does not make you think.

Then just continue to breathe regularly, with your muscles relaxed. Relaxation is a skill that requires regular practice. It's not helpful to try it for the first time when under enormous stress. Make sure you're in a quiet place and, if you have to, put ear plugs over your ears and an eye pillow over your eyes.

With practice, the Relaxation Response technique can provide the added benefit of reducing your heart rate and blood pressure, while pulling the stress out of your body. It can make a huge difference in just a short amount of time.

Meditation

Meditation is a difficult topic to tackle in such a small book. It carries many different meanings and can mean something different depending on the context or reference point. Meditation has been practiced since ancient times, but it has been more thoroughly studied and practiced for the last half a century.

Meditation is still commonly misunderstood. Many believe meditation practice has to attach itself to religious practice, but nothing is further from the truth. Meditation is generally

Stop Stressing Me Out

an inwardly oriented, personal practice that individuals do by themselves. You are generally training your mind or creating a mode of consciousness, and inside or outside of that state you realize some type of benefit.

Many people say, "I would love to mediate. I just can't sit still long enough," or "I can't turn my mind off," or "How do you sit and think about nothing? My mind races and my thoughts take over," or "My body hurts when I meditate. I can feel every ache and pain in my body when I sit still."

Just as breath work techniques come in many shapes and sizes, so does meditation. There are literally dozens of styles of meditation techniques. I like to keep things simple and divide meditation into two categories: active meditation and passive meditation.

Active meditation involves visualization, which is discussed in more detail later. You create an image, outcome, or goal in your mind, and you focus on it. You see yourself in the state that you are visualizing.

For example, if you see yourself starting and running a successful business, you create a mental picture or video of yourself doing each task and being that successful business owner. You see yourself living the life that your goal will create, and feeling the feelings and emotions that your goal will create.

Passive meditation is a process in which you ask and receive answers or guidance from your intuition, from the Universe, from GOD, a higher power, or source that you look to for information. It can be accomplished in short sessions, such as taking a brief moment of silence to clear your mind and ask the question. It can be done in longer sessions, such as formal meditation for 30-minute to one-hour intervals.

This type of meditation can be done while you sleep or take a short nap. Simply ask your question or think of your issue before sleeping, relax and breathe, let the issue go, and fall asleep. The answer will usually come to you in your sleep as an image, a phrase, a gut feeling, or a distinct situation or story.

Chapter 7: Solution # 4: Breath of Life—Deep Breathing, Meditation, and Relaxation Strategies

Meditation has been used for various health problems, such as anxiety, stress, pain, depression, insomnia, and physical and emotional symptoms associated to chronic diseases. If you suffer from any of these, try meditation. It may help and also create a sense of overall wellness.

Progressive Muscle Relaxation

This technique helps you focus on each muscle and become familiar with the sensation of relaxing your entire body. You can start from your head and work your way to your toes.

Exercise

Tense your facial muscles by biting down and furrowing your brow. Hold the tension for five to 10 seconds, then quickly release it. Next, tense your shoulder muscles by shrugging your shoulders and tucking in your chin. Hold the tension for five to 10 seconds, then release it. After that, tense your arm muscles by making a fist. Hold the tension for five to 10 seconds, then quickly release it. And so on.

Simply continue to tighten a muscle group and then release it until you have worked all the way down your body. Mentally imagine the tension evaporating as you release your tension in each muscle. Focus on the warmth and heaviness of your body parts as they relax.

The progressive muscle relaxation technique is amazing to increase body awareness and help you physically relax very quickly. If you tend to find it difficult to fall asleep at night or are fidgety, this will help you wind down fast. It also offers the added benefit of reducing muscle pain.

Visualization

Where is your happy place? A place you remember from your past, or your imaginary place that makes you feel good, feel happy, feel youthful, or relaxed when you envision it.

It can be anywhere in nature, such as the forest or the mountains, or it might be more specific, such as a cabin on a lake at a summer camp you visited as a child. It also might be an image of a beautiful place that you have never visited, such as Machu Pichu.

Exercise

Think of that place. How do you feel there? Focus on all five senses—what you would see, feel, hear, taste and smell. Allow whatever thoughts you have to pass through your mind without actually "thinking" about them.

Breathe slowly and deeply until you feel relaxed. Continue to visualize yourself there for five to 10 minutes. Then gradually return your focus to the room you are in and end the visualization.

Visualizing a pleasant place or situation is a good way to remove yourself mentally from a stressful situation. You can also use visualization in short bursts of time through-out the day to create your day or redirect negative thoughts. You can do visualization standing, sitting, or lying down, and it can be combined with other techniques such as meditation or progressive muscle relaxation.

Journaling: Release Your Stress on Paper

It has been well documented that journaling or writing about stressful experiences, similarly to talking about them, can:

- Improve immune function.
- Reduce doctor visits.
- Increase a sense of well-being.

Journaling has also been shown to help reduce the symptoms of common diseases such as asthma and rheumatoid arthritis, and help people stick to difficult programs and improve results, such as weight loss and smoking-cessation programs.

There are other journaling techniques used to release negative people and situations from your everyday thought process. You can journal then use cleansing techniques such as burning the paper, dispersing the ashes in the water, ripping the paper up an throwing in the trash, etc. By saying a statement of release, you can let go of the things that bind you to the stressor.

Chapter 7: Solution # 4: Breath of Life—Deep Breathing, Meditation, and Relaxation Strategies

It Ain't So Bad: Deflate the Danger of Your Fears

Have you experienced someone in the middle of a stressful situation completely overreacting, and been unable to change their behavior? I'm sure this has happened to everyone. The next time you feel yourself in the midst of a stressful situation, stop for a moment and look closely at your reaction and thoughts.

Is it as bad as it seems? Can the reaction to the situation be dialed down a notch or two? Does the situation really merit as much stress as you feel?

Ask these questions:

- Is there a worse possible outcome that can develop from the situation?

- Do you think that worse possible outcome will happen? If so, how likely is it?

- How would this worse possible outcome change your life?

- Is there anything else you can do to influence the result, or have you done all that is possible?

Answering these questions can help free you from stress you cannot avoid—or at minimum help you control or diminish it. In hindsight, it's never as bad as it seems when you're in the midst of it. Stop, take a deep breath, and count to 10.

Counseling to the Rescue

When all else fails and the stress-reduction techniques aren't helping, try seeking professional help. No, this does not mean you're crazy. Really, I think counseling is more misunderstood than meditation. Counseling is offered in so many ways and provides so much benefit, such as:

- How to cope with stressful conditions with less difficulty.

- How to be more effective handling conflicts, managing anger, or simply communicating with other people.

- How to resolve some of the problems that are causing you stress.

Therapy teaches you coping skills, such as cognitive restructuring, a technique that seeks to change negative thoughts and beliefs and encourage positive ones. Typically, the therapist works with you to examine and change the statements you make to yourself about your expectations and how you evaluate a situation for yourself.

Or you might want to talk to a therapist who can meet with you and your spouse, child, or coworker if the relationship is a stressful one. Or maybe you just need an impartial person to bounce your thoughts off of.

My patients tell me all the time that they feel better simply by getting things off their chest, even without any formal natural treatment or therapies. They frequently say, "I'm telling you things that I've never told anyone before." Holding your thoughts and emotions inside can cause stress and illness.

For more techniques and specific exercises you can do to practice breath work, meditation, and the other techniques discussed in this chapter, log on to www.StopStressingMeOut.com and you'll find freebies to download to help you Stop Stressing Out.

Chapter 8

Solution #5:
Exercise, It Does a Body Good—or Maybe Not?

"There is more to life than increasing its speed."
~ Mohandas K. Gandhi

I think you will agree that in today's society people don't move their bodies as much as they used to. People are more sedentary now than ever in the past, and that trend doesn't seem to be changing for the better.

There are many factors that contribute to sedentary lifestyles. Some of these include watching excessive amounts of TV, long hours sitting in front of a computer screen, working longer hours in offices, people working more jobs that are more intellectually challenging (as opposed to physically challenging).

Children are also getting significantly less movement. Children don't go outside to play as much as they used to, choosing to play video games, and sitting in front of the computer and television more often. Also, many schools have abandoned outside recess, and reduced or eliminated physical education class.

People drive more often than they walk, take the elevator more than they take the stairs, and spend more time indoors. Is technology to blame for these changes? Maybe, but it's still up to each person to get adequate exercise. If your activities of daily living have been significantly reduced due to many factors including technology, you can start exercising.

Can Exercise Harm You?

Suppose I told you that exercise could be bad for you. Suppose I asked you to stop going to the gym and driving yourself crazy trying to keep up with the latest exercise fad. Supposed I asked you to consider slowing down your current exercise routine and erasing your guilt. Would you believe that I was helping you or just telling you what you so desperately have been waiting to hear?

I'm here to validate you today. Yes, I want you to stop and take heed for a moment, so you can learn about the negative affects intense exercise can have on your body if you are stressed and burned out.

Does this sound familiar? "I'm too tired to get out of bed, how am I gonna exercise for 45 minutes?" "I'm wiped out after exercise and I don't get my energy back until two or three days later." "My personal trainer thinks I don't try hard enough, but I am trying. I just can't push myself any harder. My body's not responding."

Should exercise make you feel worse? No, but, it can. Exercise can reduce stress; however, exercise can also increase stress on the body, which is detrimental to anyone struggling with adrenal fatigue.

Chapter 1 (The Age of Stress: Today's New Silent Epidemic) discussed the effect of cortisol on the body and how the adrenal glands release cortisol during times of stress. Exercise is not widely thought of as stress, but it is. And it causes cortisol and epinephrine (adrenaline) to increase, which drains the adrenal gland.

Unfortunately, most people are told to exercise through their stress, but if the adrenal glands are fatigued intense exercise can actually be detrimental to the body and your exercise routine could actually be bad for you.

Exploring the negative effects exercise can have on the body is just as important as exploring the positive effects.

And knowing what stage of adrenal fatigue you may be in really makes a difference in the type of exercise that works best for you.

Ahhh…. Don't you feel better? Validation—it's great, isn't it?

Does this information give you permission to sit on the couch

Chapter 8: Solution # 5: Exercise, It Does a Body Good—or Maybe Not?

and eliminate exercise from your list of stress-reduction solutions? Absolutely not!

It's best to get checked out by a naturopathic physician who understands how to assess adrenal function properly. It will help you determine how your adrenals are functioning before embarking on your next exercise journey. It could save you a lot of time, money, and peace of mind.

(Stay tuned. A discussion of how to test your adrenals is discussed in Chapter 10 (Solution #7: Naturopathic Medicine: Health Care's Best Kept Secret).)

Exercise 1.0

Does this sound familiar? "I have been working out for months now and I changed my diet, but I'm not losing any weight." Many people tackle extremely intense exercise programs without understanding that they could actually be doing their body harm.

There's no law that says exercise needs to be intense in order to help you relieve stress, lose weight, or get healthy. You have to carefully choose the type of exercise that will work for your current health state and goals. If you feel burned out or drained the day after your workout, consider adjusting the type and intensity of your workout. You should feel energized after your work out and completely functional the day following.

As a stress reliever, exercise is wonderful. It can really help release stress quickly. Here are a few simple stress-relieving activities:

- Walking
- Hiking
- Yoga
- Slow endurance-type exercise
- Just being outside
- Working around the yard
- Reading before bed (something mild of course; no horrors stories or thrillers, please)

Once you've been tested and your adrenals are healthy and ready to go, then try some of these techniques; listed here are exercise specifics and guidelines to help release stress from your body:

- Basic workout outline
- Aerobic and anaerobic exercise
- The FIT principle
- Abdominal awareness
- Exercising for fat burning

Follow these recommendations for stress relief.

Basic Workout Outline

- Warm-up
- Workout period
    o Aerobic/cardiovascular training and/or
    o Anaerobic/strength training
- Cool-down

Warm-Up

The warm-up is a transition period from rest to work. Its intent is to prime your body for exercise. It's a balanced combination of light to moderately intense aerobic exercise and stretching.

The warm-up increases core body temperature, heart rate, and blood flow to your muscles and lubricates your joints—all of which enhance your exercise performance and reduce your chance of injury. Common warm-up activities include stretching, walking, jogging, or cycling for five to 10 minutes.

Aerobic Exercise (Cardiovascular)

Aerobic exercise is defined as any activity that uses large muscle groups, is maintained continuously, and is rhythmic in nature. It's the type of exercise that causes your heart and lungs to work harder than at rest.

Chapter 8: Solution # 5: Exercise, It Does a Body Good—or Maybe Not?

Aerobic activity trains your cardiovascular system to process and deliver oxygen more quickly and efficiently to your cells. Activities that require oxygen or energy for long periods of time are considered aerobic. The following are some examples of aerobic activities:

- Brisk walking
- Running
- Bicycling
- Swimming
- Skating
- Athletic dance
- Hiking
- Rowing
- Stair climbing
- Elliptical machines
- Cross-country skiing
- Jump roping

Anaerobic (Strength Training)

Any well-rounded exercise program should include strength training, which is done to increase your lean body mass and strength. Increasing lean body mass increases your basal metabolic rate, and an increased metabolic rate improves your fat-burning efficiency.

In addition, improved strength enhances your ease of performing activities of daily living and decreases your chance of injury. In order to increase strength, the muscle must be progressively overloaded by working against gradually increasing resistance.

In healthy adults, a strength-training program consists of

Stop Stressing Me Out

exercises that work all major muscle groups in a moderately intense manner. General guidelines are one to three sets of eight to 12 repetitions per exercise performed at least two days a week. It is recommended that you rest 30 to 60 seconds between sets. The following are examples of anaerobic (strength-training) exercises:

- Bench press
- Lat pull-down
- Overhead press
- Seated row
- Bicep curl
- Triceps curl
- Squat or leg press
- Leg extension
- Leg curl
- Abdominal crunch

Cool-Down

The cool-down period provides a transition for your body from work back to rest. A cool down is a rhythmic, low-intensity aerobic activity (similar to warm-up activities) for five to 10 minutes. The cool-down period helps remove lactic acid and other metabolic waste products from your working muscles, decreasing the amount of post-workout soreness and cramping you may experience. It also helps prevent blood pooling in your legs, which can cause lightheadedness and fainting.

The end of the cool-down period is the best time to increase flexibility and range of motion, which can lower your risk of injury. Stretching before and especially after you exercise has been shown to not only reduce risk of injury, but also decrease soreness after working out, enhancing muscle and joint recovery.

Chapter 8: Solution # 5: Exercise, It Does a Body Good—or Maybe Not?

This involves slow stretching of the joint to the point of slight discomfort and holding that position for 10 to 30 seconds without bouncing or straining. Stretching all your major muscle and joint groups is recommended.

The FIT Principle

The FIT principle can be used as a guideline for incorporating healthful aerobic activity as it addresses *frequency (F), intensity (I),* and *time (T)*. The following are general recommendations for healthy adults:

Frequency = the number of times per week. The minimum suggested is three times per week.

Intensity = either heart rate or perceived level of exertion.

- Heart rate (HR) = the number of heart beats per minute.

- Target HR zone = the number of heart beats per minute (your exercise intensity), measured as a percentage of maximum heart rate (Max HR).

   Aerobic benefit is generally considered to occur between 60 and 85 percent of max HR, depending on your fitness goals and physical conditioning. Exercising above that rate tends to become anaerobic.

- Max HR = theoretical maximum heart rate you can achieve during physical activity. Estimated as 220 minus your age.

   Perceived level of exertion = subjective measure of exercise intensity based on your perceived level of effort. This is often described on a scale of 1 to 10, where 10 is your maximal possible intensity. The recommended range is generally from 6 to 8. A rule of thumb is that you should exercise at a pace that allows you to carry on a conversation while exercising.

- **Time** = the length of your exercise session. The minimum recommended is usually at least 20 minutes. However, it has been shown that any activity that moderately elevates HR and breathing rate above your resting HR, for at least 10 minutes, provides some aerobic benefit.

In sum, to increase your cardio-respiratory fitness and decrease your stress, you should exercise for 20 to 60 minutes of continuous activity three to five times per week. The intensity should range from 60 to 85 percent of your maximum heart rate (max HR).

Working Your Core: Abdominal and Back Exercising

No one would argue that the abdominal or stomach area takes the prize for being a problem area for most people, and for this reason it's usually the best place to start if you are considering working only one or two body parts. A flat, tight abdominal area has been shown to have a huge health impact, as well as improve self-body image perception.

The stomach or abdominal area is a favorite place for fat to accumulate as a result of stress. Weak back muscles are also a contributing factor to increased abdominal girth. But everyone can't get down on the floor and do a million crunches a day. So, how does anyone begin the overwhelming journey of reducing his or her abdomen?

Abdominal and back exercises are listed as anaerobic exercises, so follow the basic workout plan outlined above. But if you want to begin working toward a trimmer waistline without the stress and strain of crunches, try the abdominal awareness exercise that follows.

Abdominal Awareness

Here's a little secret that will help you engage your stomach muscles automatically. Wear a belt *under* your clothing. It should be a thin and comfortable belt—the stretchy exercise belts are best—but make it tight enough so that you know it is there. The belt should fit unnoticeably under your clothing, on your bare skin.

Wearing the belt will remind you to begin using your own natural muscles to hold in your abdominal area. If you decide to wear a belt this way and learn to use it as a reminder to pull in your

Chapter 8: Solution # 5: Exercise, It Does a Body Good—or Maybe Not?

stomach, then once you start exercising your abdominal area you'll be ahead of the game.

You will have acquired "ab awareness." You will have acquired the habit of flexing or controlling your stomach muscles, and the simple act of flexing or holding in the stomach helps to tighten muscles.

Exercise and Fat-Burning

A very interesting yet rarely understood fact of exercise is that the calories burned during exercise are very few. Exercise inhibits the fat-making and fat-storing hormone insulin.

Insulin causes your cells to absorb carbohydrates (sugar) as fuel and convert the rest to fat and cholesterol. So, eating a large amount carbohydrates just before, during, or after you exercise will prevent the fat-burning effects of exercise. Protein is a better option.

Aerobic exercise burns fat while you exercise and afterward for the first 20 to 30 minutes. On the other hand, intense, high-pulse-rate (anaerobic) exercise does not burn fat during the exercise, but triggers fat-burning hormones 14 to 48 hours later.

Intense anaerobic exercise triggers several fat-burning hormones. However, if the adrenal glands are fatigued or exhausted, intense exercise can prevent weight loss and fewer fat burning hormones will be released. If your adrenals are stressed, try light aerobics (low pulse rate, endurance type), if any at all, until you get your energy back and your sleep is improved.

More Important Exercise Tips

1. Protect the spine by keeping it in a neutral position.

2. Learn proper technique and never sacrifice form for increased weight.

3. Move slowly and with control through the entire range of motion.

4. Quality over quantity every time. The more mental you make the movements, the better quality the workout.

This means to be mindful, rather than mindless, during movement training.

5. Breathe out (exhale) when exerting the most amount of effort during the movement. This usually means to breathe out during the push portion of the exercises (e.g., bench press, leg press) and breathe out during the pull portion of pull exercises (e.g., pull downs, seated row).

6. Balance the muscle groups doing the work to promote proper posture.

7. During the first week, keep resistance light and work on your technique.

8. Major or primary muscle exercises work the bigger muscles and involve the movement of more than one joint. Isolation exercises move only one joint. It is more effective to emphasize the primary movements more (and earlier in the workout) than the isolation movements. If time is short, do only primary movements.

9. Pick a weight that will allow you to go as heavy as you can to complete the desired reps but does *not* force you to lose your form and posture. If you can do two or more reps higher than the max number of reps, then you may need to go heavier.

10. Rest muscles 48 hours before working them again.

Hopefully, this chapter provided some insights as to how, when, and why it's important to exercise. But hopefully it also provided just as much insight as to why it might be best (for the time being) not to exercise.

The body needs to move, but if you're burned out and stressed, stop and evaluate before you stress even more. Stop trying to push past your intuition. You know what's best for you, and when your intuition feels a little cloudy, call a naturopathic physician and have your adrenals tested. Exercise should be beneficial and fun!

Chapter 9

Solution #6
Relax, Relate, Relieve: Melt Your Stress Away

*"Some of the secret joys of living
are not found by rushing from point A to point B,
but by inventing some imaginary letters along the way."*
~ **Douglas Pagels,** *These Are the Gifts I'd Like to Give to You*

Sleep

Sleep deprivation is on of the most under-diagnosed problems of our modern society. Seven to nine hours of sleep per day is preferable, especially for the proper functioning of the body. Yet I hear people say all the time, "I only need four or five hours of sleep. I've been that way all my life." Most people suffer from insomnia or sleep deprivation and they don't even know it.

Lack of sleep can not only lead to serious health consequences, but also jeopardize your safety and the safety of those around you. Sleep deprivation is linked to obesity, diabetes, heart disease, depression, irritability, substance abuse, increased motor vehicle accidents, decreased reaction time to signals, and problems remembering new information.

Irritability and mood swings are symptoms high on the list caused by lack of sleep. Have you ever picked a fight with your spouse for seemingly no reason? That reason could be that you were tired from lack of sleep! What about trying to remember where you put your car keys? Memory significantly decreases with each lost hour of sleep.

Sleep needs vary depending upon age, lifestyle, and health status. But the lifestyle factors that affect sleep quality and quantity, like stress and work/family schedule, have to be considered when determining your sleep needs.

Many things happen while you sleep, which makes long, good-quality sleep essential. Sleep helps:

- Growth and development. Children and adults need sleep for the necessary growth and development. Children need much more sleep than adults.

- Nervous system repair and regeneration.

- Memory, learning, and social processes, so the brain can encode and store recently received information. Sleep deprivation makes people less effective at learning new skills, and retaining or recalling recently learned information.

- Body maintenance, cell growth, and cell and tissue repair.

- The immune system to function effectively. Lack of sleep weakens the immune system, and can make you vulnerable to infection and disease. During deep sleep your body's cells increase production while proteins break down at a slower rate.

Here are a few sleep tips that will improve adrenal health. Choose a few to incorporate into your lifestyle. Just adding one or two of them will help tremendously:

- **Wear an eye pillow to keep the room as dark as possible.** Even the slightest bit of light in the room while you sleep can reduce your sleep quality.

- **Sleep in until 9:00 a.m. whenever possible.** If you can sleep just a few hours later in the morning it will help strengthen your adrenal glands.

Chapter 9: Solution # 6: Relax, Relate, Relieve: Melt Your Stress Away

- **Set a regular bedtime.** This creates a cycle and rhythm that will help your body wind down/relax easier at night.

- **Wake up at the same time every day.** This creates a cycle and rhythm that will help your body begin and maintain its daily functions more naturally and easily. It also helps you plan your day more effectively, which ultimately can lead to less stress.

- **Nap to make up for lost sleep.** If you can take a power nap during the day, please do so. Fifteen minutes a day can help you recharge and rest your body functions so they work more efficiently.

- **Be smart about napping.** If you must nap, do it in the early afternoon, and limit it to 30 minutes. Napping can interrupt your natural sleep patterns and reduce your quantity and quality of sleep.

- **Fight after-dinner drowsiness.** Try to stay awake after dinner until your actual bedtime. Napping after dinner will prevent you from falling asleep at your regular bedtime, thus reducing your amount and quality of sleep.

Rest

"There's never enough time to do all the nothing you want."
~ ***Bill Watterson,*** *Calvin and Hobbes*

Do you push yourself all day—working, commuting, taking care of the family—and then simply pass out at bedtime? Do you have a similar routine of running around all weekend completing the tasks you didn't accomplish during the week? Are you the person who falls asleep minutes after sitting down to watch TV or a movie? You just can't keep your eyes open long enough to see the end of a movie.

If so, you need rest and relaxation. When do you stop and take a deep breath? But you say, "I get my rest. I sleep five to six hours a night." That's good that you're sleeping every night, although I would like you to sleep a little longer. Five to six hours a night is a good start, but when do you actually rest? Resting and sleeping are not the same thing.

Taking time throughout the day to rest and gather your thoughts, especially just before and after meals, is valuable. Meditation and/or moments of silence or prayer are excellent for completely resting the mind and body, and should be scheduled into your daily routine, at least 30 minutes per day. The best times may be early morning before your daily routine, after work, or just before bed.

A good rule is to take a rest when you're tired. I know what you're saying, "I don't have time to rest," "There's always something else waiting for me to do when I finished the last task," "My work is never done," or (my favorite) "I rest when I go on vacation."

Well, there's no harm—only good, in fact—if you take five or 10 minutes of rest in between tasks. As a matter of fact, it's likely that the focus and peace of mind you achieve by resting just a few minutes will help you complete your next task more efficiently and quickly.

Another good tip is to take five- or 10-minute rests at select times throughout the day. For example, schedule five minutes before each meeting at work, or sit in the car for a few minutes to rest before you leave the house or once you get to work. Take five minutes to rest right before lunch. You'll be surprised by how rejuvenating a few minutes rest can be. Also, take five as soon as you walk into the house from work, but don't lie down; you may fall asleep.

Rest and sleep are two of the most important things you can do to help your adrenal glands heal. Remember: The adrenals are the stress glands, and if they aren't given the chance to heal they can become fatigued. This was discussed in Chapter 1 (The Age of Stress: Today's New Silent Epidemic).

The adrenal glands respond to rest in an amazing way. But the

Chapter 9: Solution # 6: Relax, Relate, Relieve: Melt Your Stress Away

key is that it has to be *true* rest. That means you need to lie down, and turn off the TV and other stimulating things. As mentioned in Chapter 1 (The Age of Stress: Today's New Silent Epidemic), many things in your environment create stress but are viewed as everyday activities. Watching TV, talking on the phone, listening to stimulating music, noise, etc. will ramp up your adrenal glands, not rest them.

When do you rest? Resting daily is the easiest and least expensive thing you can do for yourself to reduce stress and improve your health. You'll see immediate results. Take time, every day, several times a day to *just be*. You'll be glad you did.

Play: Have Fun!

Take time to play every day. Enjoy family and friends (play together). Take time for hobbies, recreation, and loved ones. Enjoy!

When you were a kid, your imagination used to run wild: making up games, daydreaming, imagining what life would be like as an adult. Once the reality of adulthood took over, the imagination disappeared. The good news is that your imagination is just dormant in your mind; it's not gone. You can wake it up.

If you can begin to let go and play again—I mean really let go—you won't believe how much stress you can release. And not only will the general stress reduce, but the inevitable stress in your life—the unavoidable, everyday stress—will appear less significant. Things never seem or appear as bad after you play a little.

Socialize

Humans are social creatures by nature. You need other people, particularly during stressful times. Having supportive friends, family members, and colleagues is one of the most significant ways to reduce stress.

There can't be a discussion about socializing without including technology. Technology has improved social interaction by helping people keep in touch when it would be otherwise impossible and by allowing you to have immediate interaction (for example, Skype, FaceTime, social networks, cell phones, texting, etc.).

Yet, on anther hand, technology can limit or significantly reduce our social interaction. Networking used to be done face-to-face, looking directly into peoples' eyes. Relationships were built by spending time with one another and really getting to know them. Nowadays, people substitute personal connection for artificial connection and it's not the same thing.

People need to get out of the house, out from in front of the computer, and connect with their friends and acquaintances directly—to feel their energy, emotions, and excitement. There's a time and place for both types of connection (face-to-face and technological). The key is to balance them so you don't become devoid of direct, personal contact. Everyone needs it.

Take on a Hobby, Sport, or Activity

Discussing your difficulties with someone you trust helps relieve stress and may also help you begin to solve your problems. Or you may prefer to participate in a larger social activity, such as a sports team, a spiritual group, or a group that gathers around a common interest in a hobby or some other pursuit.

These types of stress-relieving activities are often the first things to go when your schedule gets tight and your stress is too high. Yet, ironically, you are taking away one of the very things that will help you handle stress more easily. Do your best to maintain your extracurricular activities. They are better for you than you think.

Laughter

It's said that laughter is the best medicine. Laughter can reduce your blood pressure, reduce pain, reduce healing time, help prevent disease, etc. Without going into the technical inner workings of the human mind and body, we know that laughter relieves stress and just makes you feel better. We don't need a scientific study to prove that.

Chapter 9: Solution # 6: Relax, Relate, Relieve: Melt Your Stress Away

Laugh several times per day. Go see a good comedy show or film. Laughing will help you express your tensions and forget your concern for a moment. The *positive* will have replaced the *negative*.

Vacations/Stay-Cations

Vacations are interesting. Have you ever gone away to an exotic beach or location for vacation—somewhere you've been waiting to go for a long time—and by the time you arrived you were so tired you slept away the entire first day? Then it took two more days to get the stress out of your body. By the time you were in full relaxed mode three or four days of your vacation were gone, and you only had a few days left to really let go and enjoy yourself.

If so, you're not alone, except for those people who don't get the opportunity to take long vacations, by themselves or away from the family. Being guilty of waiting to rest and relax until you actually take vacation is a common theme in this society. Don't fall into the trap. Schedule vacations/stay-cations every year, but don't forget to rest and sleep daily, and to have fun regularly. It doesn't matter whether you are alone or with others, because you know how to create a blissful environment anywhere, right?

Have fun. What's life but to be enjoyed? When your troubles are mounting, go do something you love. It's hard to be stressed when you're enjoying yourself. So whether it's dinner with friends, watching a favorite movie, or taking a bubble bath, remember to make fun part of your routine.

Here are some quick tips that I find helpful. These are additional stop-stressing tips. You can implement one each day.

31 Secrets to Stop Stressing Out

- While breathing slowly in an isolated and dark place, massage your temples delicately while closing your eyes. A mild drowsiness can invade you, and a few seconds of peace can enable you to calm down.

Stop Stressing Me Out

- Take a good foam bath, listen to soft music, and use some candles to lighten around, preferably in the evening. You will be able to sleep like a baby.

- Turn your phone to silent mode, choose a good book, and settle comfortably into an armchair or in your bed. In this way you can forget your worries.

- Do not dwell over the past, source of regrets. Do not think of the future or source of anxiety. Stay in the present like children and you will avoid useless concern.

- Do not make your life move like a jet plane. Slow down.

- Do not be a slave to what the others think or say. Be a bit egoistic and please yourself.

- Know how to say no from time to time without feeling guilty. You are not considered to be better when you agree to everything. On the contrary, you will be respected and listened to much more while maintaining your sanity.

- Do not live in disorder. A pleasant and tidy environment will cheer you up more than disorder.

- If you have the possibility, long walks in the countryside or in the forest with fresh air will help you forget about everything and clarify ideas. Only the presence of your pet is authorized.

- Do not do anything that you do not want to or feel like doing. Putting something off until later does not necessarily bring misfortune. On the contrary, sometimes it is necessary to leave time to time, and then all goes back into order.

- Be positive and surround yourself with trustworthy people with whom you can talk without aggressiveness.

- Eliminate the energy robbers (things or people in your life that *drain* your energy).

Chapter 9: Solution # 6: Relax, Relate, Relieve: Melt Your Stress Away

- Eat in a calm, relaxed environment. Eating on the run can cause digestive problems. Take time to chew thoroughly; taste and smell the aromas. Don't eat and work. Take a break, relax, and enjoy your meal. Put your eating table by a window. Then sit at the table and nature watch. It's a fantastic stress-buster.

- Do one thing at a time. Resist multitasking. Trying to do too many things simultaneously inherently causes tension. Prioritize, and then calmly and efficiently go down the list.

- Attend to your financial health. Financial stress can be insidious, affecting your emotions, sleep, and physical well-being. Work out a budget to manage your expenses so that you know what your bills total and how you will pay them. If your income fluctuates, be sure you are saving enough during the higher months to cover the lean ones. Make sure your nest egg is large enough to cover unexpected expenses or sudden changes in employment. (This is usually six - eight months expenses kept in cash in the bank.) Having a plan and knowing that you are in control of your finances can go a long way toward relieving this kind of pressure.

- Be in bed before 10:00 p.m.

- Make your lifestyle a healing one.

- Believe in your ability to recover. If you can enjoy, your recovery.

- Use your mind as a powerful healing tool.

- Keep a journal. Jot down your experiences each day.

- Take the power and responsibility of your health into your own hands.

- Make whatever lifestyle changes you need to make to regain your health.

Stop Stressing Me Out

- Notice at least one small, everyday thing that you are grateful for each day.
- Look for things that make you laugh.
- Do something pleasurable every day.

Avoid:
- Getting overtired.
- Staying up past 11:00 p.m.
- Pushing yourself.
- Energy suckers.
- Being harsh or negative with yourself.
- Feeling sorry for yourself.

Chapter 10

Solution #7:
Naturopathic Medicine: Health Care's Best Kept Secret

"Let others lead small lives, but not you.
Let others argue over small things, but not you.
Let others cry over small hurts, but not you.
Let others leave their future in someone else's hands, but not you.
Not you."
~ *Jim Rohn*

After hearing all the ways you can treat stress I bet you're asking yourself, "Why don't I hear this information from my doctor when I go in for my checkup? Why am I just told that my blood pressure or stress level is too high? Why does my doctor just say to go home and take it easy? Why isn't this information given to me instead of a pill or drug?" These are very interesting questions that require good, clear explanations.

The information in this book is in alignment with the natural medicine principles that I learned while studying naturopathic medicine at Bastyr University. Naturopathic medicine is a distinct form of primary healthcare, where naturopathic physicians use traditional (old) and modern (new) approaches to focus on holistic, preventive, and comprehensive diagnosis and treatment.

In the United States, qualified naturopathic physicians undergo rigorous training before they become licensed healthcare practitioners, and the naturopathic medical profession is based on accredited educational institutions, professional licensing, national standards of practice and care, and an ongoing commitment to scientific research.

A licensed naturopathic physician (ND) attends a four-year, graduate-level naturopathic medical school and is educated in all of the same basic sciences as an MD, but also studies holistic and nontoxic approaches to therapy, with a strong emphasis on disease prevention and optimizing wellness.

In addition to a standard medical curriculum, the naturopathic physician is required to complete four years of training including clinical nutrition, homeopathy, herbal/botanical medicine, hydrotherapy, physical medicine, and counseling. Some NDs have additional training and certification in acupuncture and midwifery.

These contemporary NDs, who have attended naturopathic medical colleges recognized by the U.S. Department of Education, practice medicine as primary healthcare providers and are increasingly acknowledged as leaders in bringing about progressive changes in the nation's medical system.

You may also be wondering what the word *naturopathic* means and why you may not familiar be with it. Simply, naturopathic means the natural study and treatment of disease. What you know as common medicine today is called allopathic medicine.

Your lack of familiarity with naturopathic medicine may be because NDs and the practice of natural medicine as a licensed profession have not been generally accepted by the modern healthcare system as a legitimate medicine. Currently, only 16 states, the District of Columbia, and the United States territories of Puerto Rico and the U.S. Virgin Islands have licensing laws for naturopathic physicians.

In the past 30 years there has been an extraordinary increase in consumer demand for safe, effective, and cost-effective natural healthcare. Naturopathic medicine has emerged as the healthcare profession best suited to meet this demand.

By using protocols that minimize the risk of harm, naturopathic physicians help facilitate the body's natural ability to restore and

Chapter 10: Solution # 7: Naturopathic Medicine: Health Care's Best Kept Secret

maintain optimal health. NDs treat all medical conditions, and can provide both individual and family healthcare.

Among the most common ailments they treat are stress-related conditions, adrenal fatigue, allergies, asthma, chronic pain, diabetes, hypertension, digestive issues (like IBS, Crohn's and ulcerative colitis), female and male disorders, hormonal imbalances, weight loss/obesity, arthritis, ADHD and children's conditions, heart disease, fertility problems, menopause, cancer, skin conditions, anti-aging, fibromyalgia, and chronic fatigue syndrome.

Naturopathic physicians also function within an integrated framework—for example, referring patients to an appropriate medical specialist such as an oncologist or a surgeon.

Integrative partnerships between conventional medical doctors and licensed NDs are also becoming more available. The result can be a team-care approach that recognizes your need to receive the best overall treatment most appropriate for your specific medical condition.

As more states license naturopathic physicians, adding naturopathic medicine to your healthcare plan will become a common option.

The following principles are the foundation of naturopathic medical practice:

1. **The healing power of nature** *(Vis medicatrix naturae)*

2. **First do no harm** *(Primum non nocere)*

3. **Identify and find the cause** *(Tolle causam)*

4. **Doctor as teacher** *(Docere)*

5. **Treat the whole person**

6. **Prevention**

7. **Wellness**

Stop Stressing Me Out

"Stress should be a powerful driving force, not an obstacle."
*~ **Bill Phillips***

If you suspect that you need to stop stressing out, or that you are suffering from any condition related to stress, including chronic disease, the principles and techniques in this book will help you achieve significant stress reduction. Remember the *7 Solutions to Overcome Overwhelm and Conquer Disease Naturally.*

1. The Joy of Food: Food is Medicine
2. Nature's Stress Relief: The healing power of vitamins, minerals, herbs, essential oils, and water
3. Acupuncture - The Stress Reliever: No Pain...All Gain
4. Breath of Life: Deep breathing, Meditation and Relaxation Strategies
5. Exercise: It Does a Body good--- or Maybe Not?
6. Relax, relate, relieve: Melt Your Stress Away
7. Naturopathic medicine: Health Care's best Kept Secret

If your goal is to go deeper and you are requiring more specific recommendations for ways to address your condition, there are additional diagnostic and treatment recommendations you can follow.

It will be important for you to a have thorough health history completed to determine your stress level and any other conditions or factors affecting your health. If this health history is done in person, then a physical exam may also be performed. Your first visit may last up to one to two hours depending on the complexity of your case. This can be conducted in person or via phone or a video platform like Skype.

There are also diagnostic tests that will help to directly pinpoint the cause and severity of your condition, and how stress has affected your adrenal glands, your hormonal system, your nervous system, your immune system, detoxification pathways, and your digestive system.

Chapter 10: Solution # 7: Naturopathic Medicine: Health Care's Best Kept Secret

By identifying and understanding the cause of your condition, positive results are more likely to occur, which can significantly reduce your suffering by years, weeks, or months.

A customized health management strategy will be created with you after all the diagnostic information has been gathered and studied to teach you about managing your condition and improving your health. Although the diagnosis may be similar to what you would receive from an MD, finding the root problem and using an array of natural treatment strategies will be the goal of care.

Follow-up and continuity of care are essential when using natural medicine. The treatment strategies are not designed to be one-time fixes. They are based in lifestyle and behavior modification as well as a healing system; therefore, those looking for a quick fix may not be best suited for holistic care. But if you're willing and interested in taking control over your health and your life, these treatment strategies may be what you've been looking for.

This book, along with additional diagnostic information and treatment, could help you if:

- You're struggling with the condition and other treatments are not working.

- You have been taking medication for months or years with no real change in your health status.

- Your health seems to be declining year after year and no one, not even your doctor, understands why.

- You're exhausted or fatigued and a good night's sleep doesn't help.

- You try a whole host of natural medicine techniques, supplements, and remedies, and still don't feel any better.

- You are exercising and still not losing weight.

- Your emotions fluctuate or you're more irritable than usual.

- You can't handle stress as well as you used to.
- You're suffering from aches and pains that you can't get rid of.
- You are interested in finding out if stress management can help improve your health and quality of life.
- You just want to be healthier and slow down the aging process.

Quite frankly, it has been said that all conditions can be improved with effective stress management and treatment. So, if you suffer from any particular condition, the treatment strategies in this book, and possibly further care, will do you a world of good.

What Is a Visit Like to My Office?

My new patients receive an evaluation, which includes an initial visit that is an extensive and comprehensive, lasting approximately 60 minutes. A complete health history is completed with physical exam if necessary. Labs test, including those listed here, are done, as long as they provide helpful information to rule in or out possible conditions or contributing factors.

The purpose of this visit is for you to have a clear path and steps to take to move you toward your health goals and desires. My goal as a clinician is to help you reach your health goals, and since stress is such a significant contributing factor in disease, it is very important for your stress level to be assessed and reduced.

I also provide an added benefit of providing acupuncture. I've created a very relaxing, effective method of using acupuncture to reduce stress and create balance. It's also a great stress reliever for you to get an acupuncture treatment and primary care visit in the same location.

Let's look at a few cases of adrenal and neurotransmitter imbalances. Check to see if any of these symptoms resonates with you. If so, consultation and testing may be a good next step.

Chapter 10: Solution # 7: Naturopathic Medicine: Health Care's Best Kept Secret

Case Study #1: Early Chronic Stress Response

A 35-year-old female with a "type A" personality was recently diagnosed with high blood pressure. She also has headaches, mild anxiety, and is having trouble sleeping at night. Her stress level is very high right now. She's recently divorced, and her boss has been putting pressure on her to improve her work performance, but she's been having trouble concentrating.

She's very active and athletic. She works out five days a week. She says she eats well and drinks a protein shake before each workout. She drinks alcohol a few nights a week when she's out with friends.

She had her adrenals and neurotransmitters tested with the following results:

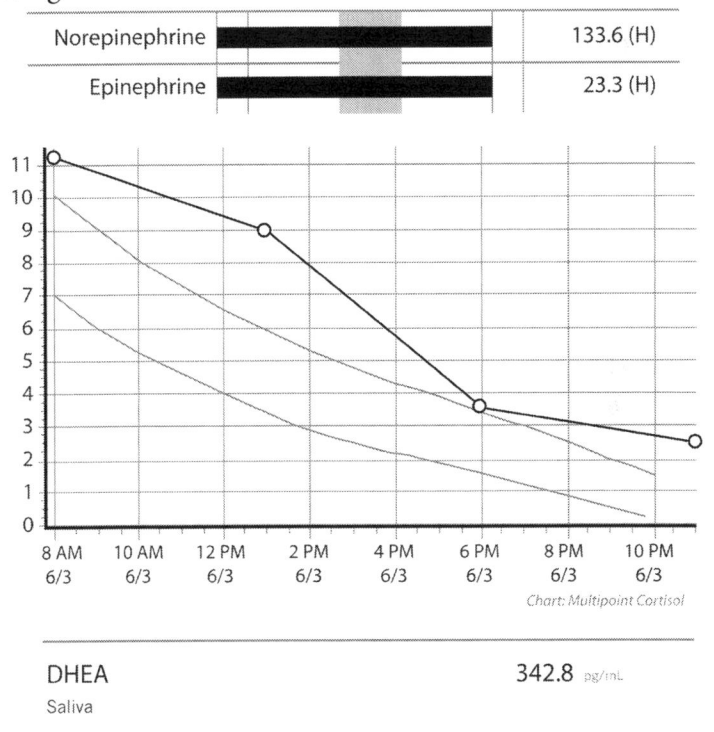

Norepinephrine	133.6 (H)
Epinephrine	23.3 (H)

Chart: Multipoint Cortisol

DHEA	342.8 pg/mL
Saliva	

Her epinephrine and norepinephrine are very high. Her cortisol levels (represented by the red dotted line) are elevated throughout the entire day and at night. But her DHEA is still in normal range.

113

Stop Stressing Me Out

This is typical early-stage adrenal fatigue, where the cortisol, norepinephrine, and epinephrine are elevated. These labs confirm why her blood pressure is high. She has anxiety and a lack of concentration, and they possibly explain why she has headaches. Her high nighttime cortisol explains why she's not sleeping well.

She's over-stimulated and would benefit from adrenal support that would calm down her adrenal glands, and reduce the output of cortisol, epinephrine, and norepinephrine. She would also benefit from an adaptogenic herb to provide support to her adrenals since they are working so hard.

Case Study #2: Mid-Stage Chronic Stress Response

A 45-year-old female states she has depression, irritability, thinning hair, and irregular menses. She has severe afternoon fatigue but has difficulty staying asleep at night. She's wired but tired. She has weight gain and describes her diet as poor diet, and she craves sugar and caffeine.

She has a high-stress job and also cares for a sick parent five days per week. She's married, but unhappily. They're contemplating divorce and they have a lot of disagreements over financial issues.

She feels like she's getting worse every year but can't pinpoint any one thing that is contributing to her decline in health. She tried dieting, but doesn't have the motivation to maintain a healthy lifestyle. She also says she has no free time to exercise.

Her adrenals and neurotransmitters were tested with the following results:

Chapter 10: Solution # 7: Naturopathic Medicine: Health Care's Best Kept Secret

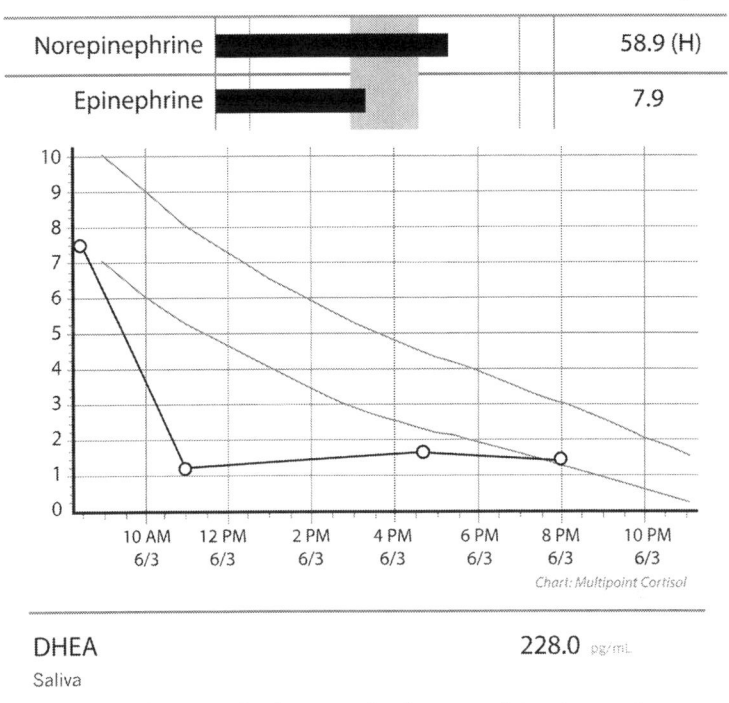

Norepinephrine	58.9 (H)
Epinephrine	7.9

Chart: Multipoint Cortisol

DHEA	228.0 pg/mL
Saliva	

Her cortisol is on the low end of normal in the early morning and evening, and low in the late morning through mid-evening. This explains why she has severe afternoon fatigue. It would have been best for her to test later in the evening to see if her cortisol started to rise at night to assess her sleep issues.

Epinephrine is normal and norepinephrine is high. This explains her depression and irritability, and why she has many mental, emotional complaints.

Her DHEA is on the low end of normal, which would also point to her sex hormones being reduced. Her sex hormones and other endocrine glands need to be tested, especially since her periods are irregular and she having hair thinning, to rule out thyroid problems. She's probably perimenopausal.

This is classic mid-stage chronic stress response. Where some results are high, others are low or normal. The classic presentation is the wired but tired feeling. This is the most common patient I see.

Her treatment plan is more of a mixed bag. Her adrenals need to be stimulated at certain times of the day and calmed at others, so it's very important for her to follow her protocol precisely. She would also benefit from an adaptogenic herb to provide support to his adrenals to help build them back up.

Additionally, she would benefit from incorporating stress-reduction techniques, since it appears that many of her stress-related activities would be difficult to change right now. Those things in your life that can't be changed or would be too difficult to change are called "obstacles to cure."

Helping her would be a step-by-step process designed not to add too much more stress to her life. She would begin with a very simple protocol. But she would begin to feel better within a few days to weeks of beginning her protocol. Lasting improvement may take some time.

Case Study #3: Late-Stage Chronic Stress Response— Adrenal Fatigue

A 52-year-old menopausal female complains of fatigue/exhaustion, hot flashes, anxiety, difficulty dealing with stress, reduced memory, headaches, weight gain, and loss of libido.

She has three children (23, 21, and 17 years old). She's a professional with a high-stress job, and the stress has been increasing each year since she started working there 12 years ago.

She has a really good diet. She eats organic, and avoids dairy, beef, and gluten due to food sensitivities. She had a past history of irritable bowel syndrome (IBS) and acne and since she began avoiding those, her IBS and acne cleared up.

She's been taking hormone replacement therapy since it was prescribed two years ago for her hot flashes and low female hormones. Her symptoms have not improved, which is why she's seeking additional treatment.

Her adrenals and neurotransmitters were tested with the following results:

Chapter 10: Solution # 7: Naturopathic Medicine: Health Care's Best Kept Secret

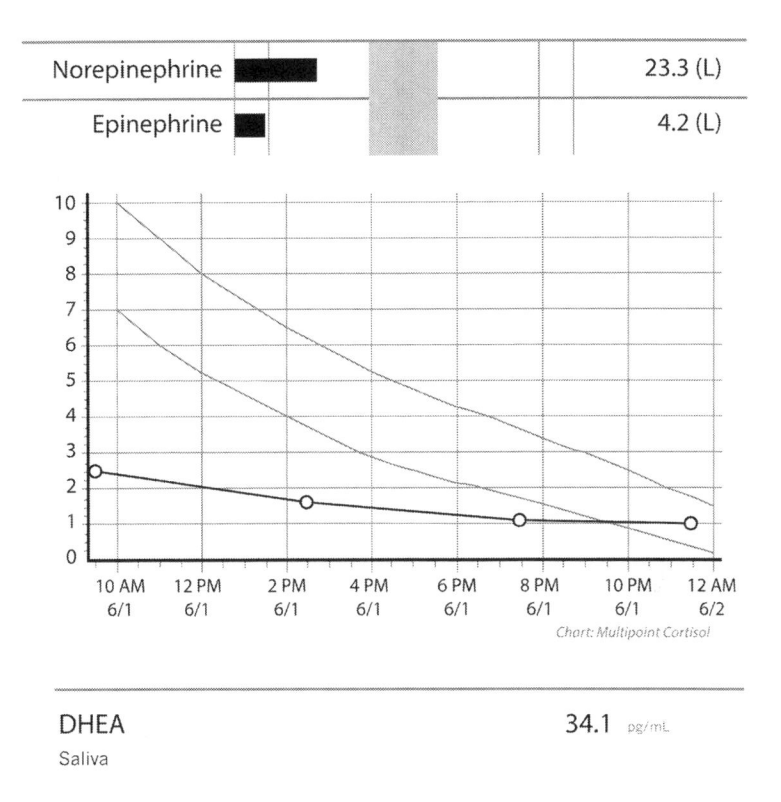

Norepinephrine		23.3 (L)
Epinephrine		4.2 (L)

Chart: Multipoint Cortisol

DHEA	34.1 pg/mL
Saliva	

All her results are very much below normal, except that her nighttime cortisol is in normal range. This is a very clear example of adrenal fatigue. It's no surprise that she's suffering from so many symptoms, especially fatigue and difficulty handling stress.

She isn't producing enough cortisol or DHEA to sustain herself. Cortisol is a very powerful natural anti-inflammatory (fights inflammation), so it's not surprising that she had IBS and struggles with food allergies.

She's having weight challenges, which are indicated by her low epinephrine and cortisol. She's also having memory problems and anxiety, which can also be deduced from her neurotransmitter levels.

A complete analysis would include additional neurotransmitters, which were tested in her case, like serotonin, GABA, glutamate, and dopamine. These results are past the scope of this book, but assessing the combination of her results would provide a great deal more insight into her other symptoms.

Since she's menopausal, it also recommended that she retest her sex hormones to ensure that the hormone replacement therapy she's currently taking is keeping her hormones within normal ranges, and to ensure her additional symptom of hot flashes do not have another cause.

If she came to me before being put on hormone replacement therapy, I would have provided adrenal support first, to improve her symptoms and possibly avoid drug therapy.

There are so many additional layers to her case, and it will take some time to maintain lasting improvements, but she is a perfect example of how complex and intricate the body is. It also helps to understand how individual assessment and treatment are necessary. The same treatment cannot be provided just because someone shows up with particularly similar symptoms.

This individualized care is the hallmark of naturopathic medicine. My favorite phrase for explaining what's special about naturopathic medicine is "Symptoms and diseases may have the same name, but they can have a different cause. Unless you treat the specific cause, healing isn't likely."

I hope this gives you an idea of what your adrenals and neurotransmitters may look like and the symptoms that go along with them. But this is still only a small portion of how you would be assessed. Additionally, there are other considerations that would be addressed over time.

Part of your care would include detoxification and dietary adjustments, supplements, acupuncture, herbs, etc. Everything is based on what's needed for your personalized health and healing. Over time the protocols are adjusted as the body improves. It's a very dynamic process.

Get your free "Stop Stressing Me Out" quiz!

"More Information and More Insight: 3 Ways to Release Your Stress Even Faster"

Take the quiz and you will:

1. See how high (or, hopefully, low) you score on the "Stop Stressing Me Out" quiz. Find out how much stress you really have.

2. Discover the physical signs and symptoms associated with stress, which signs and symptoms you have, and which specific strategies will work best for you.

3. Find out how you are actually coping with your stress on the Stressed-Out Scale. Are you a candidate for burnout, in burnout, or in adrenal fatigue?

After you take the quiz, you'll have the opportunity to talk directly with Dr. Lewis to find out what you can do to reverse the signs of stress.

The consultation is guaranteed to provide you with deeper insight into your state of stress and health. You will be inspired to move forward with additional strategies and tips to reduce your tension, live healthier, and take control of your life.

Get your free quiz at
www.StopStressingMeOut.com/quiz

Made in the USA
Charleston, SC
09 June 2014